# Intermittent
# FASTING

## — MADE EASY —

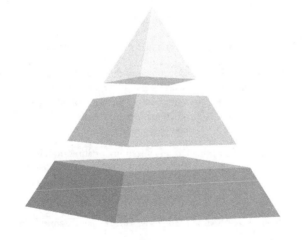

# THE 21-DAY
# PYRAMID PLAN

First Edition: November 2019

10 9 8 7 6 5 4 3 2 1

ISBN: 978-0-9992123-6-3

Cover design and formatting by

Intermittent Fasting Made Easy: The 21-Day Pyramid Plan

© 2019 by Dawna Stone

**Healthy You Ventures, LLC**

# Table of Contents

# Introduction

Intermittent fasting is taking the country by storm! It can however, be really hard to follow. After experimenting with several intermittent fasting protocols, I discovered a better way to intermittent fast. A way that makes following intermittent fasting so much easier to adhere to. But, before I get into the pyramid method, let me tell you a little about me.

I've been helping people lose weight for more than two decades. What started out as simply a way to help family (I helped my dad lose more than 70 pounds) and co-workers get fit, healthy and lose unwanted pounds became a passion for me. In 1997 while working full-time as a strategy consultant for Deloitte Consulting, I spent my free time studying for and becoming a certified health and weight loss coach. In 1998 I began formally working with people to help them lose weight. Although just a side gig, I helped numerous people in Newport Beach, California, where I opened a weight loss clinic and coached people in the evenings and on the weekends.

I have always loved helping people reach their weight loss goals. The problem for me was that I had a very demanding full-time job and I could only help a small number of people at any given time. After years of helping people whenever possible, I found a way to help a larger number of people by giving group talks, giving expert advice on radio and TV and writing for numerous websites and magazines. It felt good to be reaching and helping more and more people.

Eventually, I got a segment on FOX News called "Healthy Living with Dawna Stone" and a few years later, my own radio show on Sirius Satellite Radio called "Health and Fitness Talk with Dawna Stone." The TV segment and radio show allowed me to reach even more people and share my knowledge of health and weight loss. I was feeling great about helping so many people, but I still wanted to help more.

In 2012 after selling my two companies, *Women's Running* magazine (which I launched in 2004) and the Women's Half Marathon Series (which I launched in 2009) I decided to write a weight loss book that would help thousands more people get healthy and lose weight. The book, *Healthy You! 14 Days to Quick and Permanent Weight Loss and a Healthier, Happier You,* became an instant success and the self-published book quickly turned into a six-figure book deal for a cookbook that expanded on the *Healthy You!* concept. I was finally in a position where I was no longer helping just hundreds or thousands of people but now hundreds of thousands of people. Since then, I've written several more books and continue to do my best to help as many people as possible reach a healthy weight.

This book, The Intermittent Fasting Pyramid, is different than my other books. Most of my previous weight loss books focus on clean eating. I was even named by *Prevention Magazine* as one of the best clean eating bloggers. So you may wonder, why the change from clean eating to intermittent fasting?

Although I've helped so many people lose weight by eating clean, it's no secret that eating clean takes a great deal of effort and a lot of will power. It does get easier the longer you stick to it, but many people find the strict diet difficult to adhere to. Even I would go through stages of adhering to a clean eating diet to only fall off the clean eating bandwagon for weeks at a time.

When I discovered intermittent fasting, it was like a secret weapon against weight gain. And it was a way for me to eat some of my not-so-healthy favorite foods without slowing my weight loss or gaining weight. More importantly, I was immediately intrigued by all the positive scientific research that touted the numerous health benefits of intermittent fasting. Intermittent fasting not only helps people lose weight without having to stick to strict dieting rules for long periods of time, but it also showed numerous health benefits—we will talk more about these benefits in future chapters.

Unfortunately (yes, there is an unfortunately), as with many diet programs, I found intermittent fasting to work great initially but to get more difficult to stick to the longer I tried to adhere to the program. That is, as soon as the novelty of intermittent fasting wore off, I found it more and more difficult to continue to adhere to the diet's protocols. And even more disappointing, I found that the longer I was able to stick to intermittent fasting, the more likely I became to binge following my fasting days.

I tried many of the popular intermittent fasting programs including the Five Two diet (5:2), alternate day fasting, and the 16/8 Method.

But all of the programs that I tried had one downfall for me: the tendency for binging following my fasting days. That is, I would overcompensate following my fasting days. I knew intermittent fasting worked but I just needed to find a way for it to be easier to follow and, specifically, a way to overcome the tendency to overeat on the days following my fasting days.

Keeping all the research and medical studies in mind, I went out in search of a way to make intermittent fasting and all the benefits you get from it easier. What I discovered was that you could easily structure your intermittent fasting practice in a way that deters you from binging post fast—a structure that makes intermittent fasting easier to adhere to for the long term. And a structure that actually provides even more rapid results, keeping motivation high and success more eminent.

The secret is the intermittent fasting pyramid structure, which allows for your fasting day to be followed by two partial fasting days. The gradual increase of calories from your fasting day to your partial fasting day deters binging and supercharges weight loss.

The intermittent fasting pyramid:

- Allows for the same scientifically proven benefits of intermittent fasting but is easier to adhere to

- Deters binging after your fasting day

- Allows for more weight loss and improves health

If you are ready to try intermittent fasting but are worried about sticking to a strict intermittent fasting practice, the intermittent fasting pyramid may be just what you need. The intermittent fasting pyramid makes intermittent fasting easy!

If you are ready to reach your weight loss goals, get healthy and reap the many benefits that intermittent fasting provides, you've come to the right place.

Let's get started!

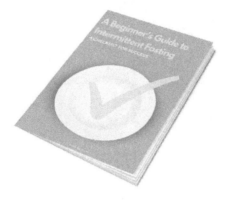

## Boost Your Success with Your FREE Intermittent Fasting Checklist!

Go to: https://dawnastone.com/guide-to-intermittent-fasting

# CHAPTER 1:

# The Intermittent Fasting Pyramid – A Better Way

*Rachel was quite familiar with intermittent fasting. In fact, she was familiar with at least a dozen different diets that she had tried over the years. But when her doctor told her that she was borderline diabetic, she was determined to make a change. Having struggled with excess weight all her life, Rachel wanted to slim down to a healthy weight. Likewise, she wanted to be healthier and choose a diet that would keep her from having to start medication for her blood sugar. Intermittent fasting was the diet she thought would be best in accomplishing this.*

*Having read a great deal about intermittent fasting, Rachel knew of many people who had not only lost weight but who had also improved their blood sugar and blood pressure on the diet. Actually, this had been one reason she had tried it in the past. But when she had tried intermittent fasting on two prior occasions, both attempts failed. The first time, she had difficulty completely fasting two days each week. And the second time, she found herself overcompensating the day after the fast. In both instances, she didn't lose weight and only became dejected and frustrated.*

*That was before she heard about the Intermittent Fasting Pyramid. Unlike other intermittent fasting plans, the Intermittent Fasting Pyramid is structured in a way that made intermittent fast-*

*ing more tolerable and less frustrating. Likewise, the program made food binges after fasting less likely by allowing a gradual transition between fasting and one's regular diet. After educating herself about the program, Rachel tried once again to incorporate intermittent fasting into her life. And with the Intermittent Fasting Pyramid, she was finally able to do so successfully.*

*Six months later, Rachel had lost over 18 pounds, had much more energy, and had kept her blood sugar in the normal range without medication. Not only did she look and feel healthier, but she no longer had a problem continuing with her intermittent fasting diet as a lifestyle choice. By choosing the Intermittent Fasting Pyramid, Rachel found intermittent fasting to be much more tolerable, allowing her to see the results she wanted. And it's a big reason why she is one of the diet's biggest proponents today.*

## The Intermittent Fasting Pyramid – An Overview

Like Rachel, many people who have tried intermittent fasting in the past have struggled to see the weight loss and health results they wanted in the long term. For some, it becomes difficult to stick to a fasting schedule because of distractions and temptations. For others, post-fasting food binges undermine the potential benefits of the diet. Though these are common struggles with intermittent fasting, this dietary approach to weight loss and health has proven advantages. Both history and science have shown that intermittent fasting is a smart approach to dieting.

The Intermittent Fasting Pyramid was designed to address the common struggles associated with intermittent fasting while empowering people to adopt this dietary strategy to become healthier. The Intermittent Fasting Pyramid, like many of today's popular intermittent fasting plans, does allow a small percentage of your daily calories to be consumed rather than requiring a complete fast. But it differs in that its structure incorporates two transitional days following your fasting day. As a result, the period of time you fast is more tolerable, and the threat of post-fast binges are less. These two features of the Intermittent Fasting Pyramid will help you succeed with your intermittent fasting practice.

In essence, the Intermittent Fasting Pyramid consists of fasting, partial fasting, and non-fasting days. You start your week (typically a Monday) with your fasting day, (Day 1), which allows you to have 25 percent of your daily calorie needs. Day 1 is then followed by two partial fasting days, (Days 2 and 3), which allow you to eat half your daily calorie needs each day. And then, the partial fasting days are followed by four non-fasting days, (Days 4, 5, 6 and 7), which allow you to eat your regular diet. Once you complete this 7-day schedule, you then simply repeat it each week, reaping the weight loss and health benefits of intermittent fasting along the way.

As you can see, the Intermittent Fasting Pyramid allows you to supercharge your weight loss by incorporating partial fasting days, which extend your fasting time for three entire days. Don't let this time frame scare you. Only one day cuts your calories to 25 percent of your caloric need. The other two days gradually increase your calories until you've reached your non-fasting days. This potentially offers greater advantages when compared to other intermittent fasting schedules because of the greater duration of moderated fasting time. And the Intermittent Fasting Pyramid provides a gradual transition back into your regular diet, which deters binge eating and overcompensation. As with other intermittent fasting programs, you should adhere to an 8-hour eating window on your fasting and partial fasting days—more on this later.

In the chapters that follow, the historical significance and scientific evidence supporting intermittent fasting will be provided, demonstrating the many ways in which intermittent fasting enhances wellness. Likewise, more detailed explanations about the Intermittent Fasting Pyramid will be covered along with how to implement this innovative intermittent fasting strategy into your life. This information will help you appreciate not only why intermittent fasting offers a healthy way to achieve the weight loss you want, but also help you understand why the Intermittent Fasting Pyramid makes it easier to realize long-term health benefits.

# Don't Do It Alone!

## Join Me For The Intermittent Fasting Pyramid Online Challenge

Want a little extra motivation to help you get started and stick to the plan? Join me and take the 3-week Intermittent Fasting Pyramid Online Challenge. With the online challenge, you will have everything you need to succeed and I will personally be your guide on this incredible journey.

Go to www.DawnaStone.com/IntermittentFasting to learn more and to sign up!

# SECTION I:

# The Beginning

# CHAPTER 2:

# The History of Fasting

When it comes to basic essentials, food is pretty high on the list right behind water. Without adequate nutrition, our bodies are unable to fight off infection and disease, and they become unable to keep things in their proper balance. Therefore, it may seem a little odd that human beings ever decided that fasting might be something beneficial. After all, even cave dwellers were likely more concerned about their next meal than they were about skipping a few meals for their overall wellness.

Considering our prehistoric relatives raises some interesting ideas about fasting. Understandably, grocery markets were not on every neighborhood corner, and opportunities for a meal were hit or miss. It was truly feast or famine. As a result, some believe that the benefits provided by fasting developed based on our evolutionary past. Because food was available only intermittently, our ancestors' bodies and metabolism had to adapt. And those who did so successfully naturally survived—passing along these metabolic preferences to future generations.

Whether or not this evolutionary aspect of fasting is real or not, fasting as a practice has been common for many centuries. Some ancient cultures adopted fasting rituals as a means to enhance spirituality. Others used fasting to promote better physical and mental health. Interestingly, the rationale behind fasting hasn't changed much over time, although we tend to have more science behind the subject. Even in ancient times, fasting was encouraged for the same reasons it is today. If nothing else, fasting has certainly stood the test of time.

In this chapter, we will explore some ancient beliefs about fasting and those who encouraged its regular use. These beliefs pertained not only to religious rituals but also to benefits associated with learning and health. And the link between these more remote rituals and today's modern fasting practices will be considered as well. In doing so, you will begin to appreciate the role fasting has played throughout our history, and you will be better able to see how fasting can actually promote better health and wellness.

## The History of Fasting and Religion

If you traditionally associate fasting with various religious practices, then you are certainly not alone. Numerous religions practice fasting as part of their spiritual rituals. For example, Buddhist tradition incorporates daily fasting in its religious practices as does Christianity, Judaism, and Islam. For centuries, these religions promoted individual fasting as a means for people to connect with their spiritual side. And collective fasting rituals, such as Yom Kippur in Judaism and Ramadan in Islam, are group-related religious traditions practiced by most followers of these religions. Thus, fasting as a means to promote spiritual wellness has been long appreciated.

From a historical standpoint, each of these religions practices fasting in slightly different ways. Some require fasting for 24 hours while others may only involve portions of the day.

Likewise, some specify certain foods and liquids that may or may not be allowed during the fast. But while these nuances are unique to each religion's specific spiritual rituals, fasting tends to be used for common purposes. These purposes primarily involve efforts directed at personal atonement to ask for divine forgiveness, and/or they involve a means to embrace a deeper sense of humility through personal suffering. In both cases, fasting offers a way for a heightened sense of spiritual awareness.[1]

The common practice of fasting among so many different religions across the globe is intriguing given the fact that these areas were generally isolated from one another. And it is unlikely that these religious practices had anything to do with weight loss or even physical health. But fasting has been associated with enhanced ability to concentrate and focus. Thus, the ability to meditate and connect with one's spiritual side is something that would be expected from a religious fast. In the spirit of holistic health, fasting can therefore be appreciated historically for the benefits it provided not only spiritually but also in mental clarity.

## The History of Fasting for Health

Fasting was not only for religious purposes. Several ancient healers and philosophers encouraged the use of fasting for wellness. One of the oldest theories of fasting was described by the Greek mathematician and philosopher Pythagoras. As an avid learner, he traveled far and wide to attain knowledge, and one of his ventures took him to Egypt. As was common practice then, Pythagoras had to fast for 40 days before he could attend the Egyptian school. Fasting was believed to enhance learning by improving one's attention and memory. Pythagoras was so impressed by the practice that he encouraged fasting among the Greeks upon his return.[2]

Of course, Pythagoras was not alone. Aristotle and Plato also encouraged regular fasting to improve health and wellness. Hippocrates believed fasting was the fastest way to overcome an illness. While eating was believed to fuel one's infection or disease, fasting was theorized to "starve" the illness and promote self-healing. Hippocrates supported his theories by noting how individuals and animals alike naturally don't feel like eating when sick. He believed that people triggered their innate healing abilities. In fact, fasting has been called "the physician within," highlighting fasting's inherent ability to promote health. Even Benjamin Franklin recognized these benefits, stating that rest and fasting offered the most effective means to stay healthy.[3] Thus, the practice of fasting in promoting wellness has a history nearly as long as its use for spiritual purposes.

In more recent times, fasting was reinvigorated as an important approach to health and wellness in the late nineteenth century. One of the medical pioneers at the time was a physician out of the University of Michigan named E.H. Dewey. It was his belief that excessive eating was the cause of many illnesses, and similarly, he recommended eating only two meals a day combined with longer fasts. Several others began studying the effects of fasting on metabolism, weight loss, and general wellness thereafter.[4] By the mid-twentieth century, many physicians and nutritionists were acknowledging the health benefits of fasting for some people.

## Fasting – From Ancient Civilizations to Modern Times

The advantages the ancient Greeks and religious cultures understood about fasting have only grown in magnitude today. Over the last several decades, an increasing amount of research has been conducted trying to determine not only the actual benefits of fasting but also the mechanisms behind these positive effects. In terms of overall health, fasting boosts some proteins in the brain that promote better thinking, attention and memory. Likewise, fasting also reduces the risk of heart disease as well as some cancers. And these health benefits are completely unrelated to weight loss.[5]

At the same time, research shows how fasting improves our ability to have a healthy metabolism and to better manage our weight. For example, when you begin fasting, your body begins creating glucose initially to compensate for the lack of food. But thereafter, fatty acids from fatty tissues begin to be used for energy. This naturally can boost weight loss and, at the same time, improve your body's ability to use glucose when it's available. Not only does this promote a healthier weight, but it also boosts your metabolism and reduces your chances of developing diabetes. This explains how fasting offers several health benefits, including weight loss, through specific effects it has on the body.

Though many of the ways that fasting promotes wellness have yet to be well defined, fasting's longstanding history substantiates its role in holistic health. Certainly, fasting has positive metabolism effects, but it is also psychologically empowering. From spirituality, to mental wellness, to weight loss, fasting's benefits have been recognized from many centuries throughout the world. Likewise, when performed properly, its history also shows that fasting is a safe way to improve wellness. By choosing fasting as a strategy, you are in excellent company based on its popularity as a wellness technique through time.

# CHAPTER 3:

# The History of Intermittent Fasting

From the previous chapter, it seems pretty clear that we, as a race, have been fasting since the beginning of mankind. What may have started out as fasting by default in our prehistoric relatives ultimately culminated in religious rituals and wellness practices. These practices have endured over the centuries and continue to play a role in spirituality. But more recently, fasting has been appreciated in a more modernized way when it comes to wellness. And while many versions of fasting exist in today's health conversations, most all use the term intermittent fasting to describe current fasting practices.

Calling fasting by the name "intermittent fasting" might seem a little redundant. After all, all types of fasting are intermittent in nature. Fasting that goes on indefinitely is not a good idea and represents a certain way to undermine your well-being as you starve yourself to death. However, the term intermittent fasting is more associated with specific regimens of fasting that have regular, periodic fasting schedules. And in actuality, the history of these more modern dietary approaches to fasting is much more abbreviated. Regardless, given the popularity and support for intermittent fasting today, exploring its recent history is also of value.

## Understanding Intermittent Fasting through Today's Lens

As discussed in the previous chapter on fasting, several researchers and physicians began to explore fasting as a therapeutic diet for weight loss and health in the nineteenth and twentieth centuries. Though the science was not as robust, evidence did support some benefits. However, fasting as a type of pervasive diet and health plan never really took hold during those years. For one, the state of science lacked adequate proof of its benefits. And more importantly, population health and social behaviors were not nearly as complex as they are today. These latter developments have actually brought dietary fasting back to the forefront of health discussions.

Consider a snapshot of today's world. Obesity is a tremendous problem globally with up to half of all adults being overweight or obese. At the same time, one in every 10 people in the U.S. have diabetes with most having concurrent weight challenges.[6] While these health conditions are due to a number of factors, diet remains a major consideration for both prevention and intervention. And because our eating habits have changed a great deal in the last century, it only makes sense that re-exploring old dietary practices might occur. In part, this helped bring fasting back into the conversation.

While the obesity and diabetes epidemics have been catalysts in reconsidering fasting as a health and diet strategy, these aren't the only ones. Other social trends are also present that encourage greater involvement in one's health and wellness. Rather than taking pills and medications, people increasingly want to participate in preventative practices and alternative, natural options of care. As a means to treat excess weight and diabetes, fasting therefore offers an approach that embraces self-empowerment and control. These social trends offer another reason why fasting has reentered the scene.

Lastly, today's healthcare enjoys a rapidly expanding environment of scientific evidence to better guide new practices. While the science behind intermittent fasting will be discussed in detail in later chapters, suffice it to say that increasing support for intermittent fasting in promoting health has also played a role in its recent popularity. Though some studies truly served as a tipping point that prompted intermittent fasting to attract widespread attention, the quantity of positive evidence between intermittent fasting and health has been progressively growing. All of these factors can be seen as impacting the recent history of intermittent fasting's rise in popularity.

## Mixing Science with Pop Culture – How Intermittent Fasting Gained Recognition

Though specific dietary trends cannot usually be linked to a single moment in time, that is not the case with intermittent fasting. The recent popularity of intermittent fasting is actually linked to the airing of a television show on the BBC network called *Horizons*. The program was entitled, "Eat, Fast and Live Longer," which was broadcast in August of 2012.[7] The show was hosted by British journalist, Michael Mosely, who explored the science behind intermittent fasting. And at the same time, performed his own self-experiment using the popular 5:2 intermittent fasting protocol.

What drove Michael Mosley to experiment with intermittent fasting at the time involved two major events. The first was scientific. Research published in the United Kingdom had recently shown how intermittent fasting had not only resulted in significant weight loss among over 100 people, but it also had reversed many of their diabetic markers.[8] The second was more personal. Mosely had recently been diagnosed with diabetes and wanted to avoid taking medication.

In addition to the BBC's program highlighting the recent evidence linking intermittent fasting to better health, Mosley's experiment was also a success. In roughly 9 weeks, he lost 20 pounds, and his lab tests no longer supported a diagnosis of diabetes. And with *Horizons* reaching millions of viewers, immediate interest in intermittent fasting was stimulated. Within a year's time, the dietary trend had grown immensely in the United Kingdom, and Michael Mosley's book, *The Fast Diet*, was an Amazon best seller.[9] Intermittent fasting soon spread to the U.S. and other countries as a promising diet that not only helped people lose weight but also enhanced overall wellness.

Though several different versions of intermittent fasting diets exist today, the recent surge in interest of these diets essentially started in 2012. Since that time, the amount of research into intermittent fasting diets has grown considerably, and new revelations about how intermittent fasting works to improve health continue to be discovered. While it is true that fasting has been recognized for centuries as being beneficial, it took a combination of popular media and new research to launch intermittent fasting back into the mainstream.

## Understanding Categories of Intermittent Fasting

Historically speaking, all intermittent fasting programs consist of cycles of regular fasting and eating periods. From this perspective, intermittent can be considered a "catch-all" term that describes periodic reductions in calories on a regular basis. Intermittent fasting has also been called intermittent energy restriction, since it cuts down calorie intake during fasting episodes. This is in contrast to most diets that are continuous calorie restriction programs.

While intermittent fasting is an umbrella term, specific types of intermittent fasting protocols are also commonly recognized. Some consist of whole-day fasting protocols where you fast for the entire day. Others protocols call for a major restriction of calories on fasting days. For example, the 5:2 intermittent fasting diet involves 5 days of regular eating with 2 days of fasting each week. The fasting days, however, do not represent complete absence of food or liquids. For example, the 5:2 intermittent fasting diet suggests less than 600 calories on your fasting days.

Other intermittent fasting diets are time-restricted diets. In these protocols, you do not fast the entire day, but instead, you restrict your eating to certain times or amounts of time during your fasting periods. An example of this type of intermittent fasting diet is the 16:8 diet. In this intermittent fasting protocol, you would only be allowed to eat during an 8-hour period each day leaving the other 16 hours for fasting. While these represent different approaches to intermittent fasting, both strategies have been shown to help with weight loss and in promoting better health.

## From History to the Present

Certainly, fasting is not new, and it has been practiced for a number of reasons throughout time. But the recent popularity of intermittent fasting has resulted from a confluence of factors that make this an attractive dietary trend. For one, intermittent fasting is often much easier than other types of diets. Because fasting is intermittent, and you are allowed to eat normally at other times, the degree of hunger you may experience is less overall when compared to diets than continuously restrict your calories. Secondly, intermittent fasting offers a much-needed solution to many of the health issues we face today in society.

One additional thing can be appreciated in considering the recent history of intermittent fasting. Change and progress are occurring at a much more rapid pace than they were even a decade ago. What we are learning now about intermittent fasting and its impact on health continues to expand as new research becomes available. This information can further help refine how to best implement an intermittent fasting program. In fact, this book seeks to do just that based on the most recent research available.

SECTION II:

# The Pyramid Explained

# CHAPTER 4:

# Welcome to the Intermittent Fasting Pyramid!

Given the history of both fasting and intermittent fasting, there's a good chance you might have already given this weight loss approach a shot. Since 2012, millions have tried intermittent fasting, and while many have succeeded in attaining their goals, others have not. With this in mind, the Intermittent Fasting Pyramid hopes to provide those that struggled with intermittent fasting a better chance of realizing the weight loss they want. And at the same time, the Intermittent Fasting Pyramid also offers those who have had success with intermittent fasting opportunities for customization and flexibility. Thus, anyone can potentially benefit from this diet and weight loss strategy.

As noted, intermittent fasting can come in a few different varieties. Some require complete restriction of all calories during a fasting day while others reduce the number of calories allowed or limit fasting hours to less than a full day. For the Intermittent Fasting Pyramid, the recommended approach is a reduced number of calories on fasting days and to limit your eating window to 8 hours which will be further outlined when the pyramid plan is detailed. Not only does this strategy reduce your frustration and degree of hunger, but it also has been shown to help you stick to your diet longer. And the longer you can stay on track, the better your chances of achieving your weight and health targets. That's what the Intermittent Fasting Pyramid has to offer!

## Another Diet Pyramid?

If you're not new to dieting, then you're likely familiar with a variety of pyramids that described different approaches to healthy eating and specific nutritional diets. In fact, the first diet pyramid was initially introduced in Sweden back in 1974. The Swedish National Board of Health wanted to publicize basic foods everyone needed that were relatively affordable at the time. Then, other more expensive food groups could be eaten less often as supplements to improve overall wellbeing. Though the national group designed something that looked more like a pie chart, one of the large retail food chains in Sweden came up with the idea of a pyramid. Since a pyramid's base is naturally wider than its peak, foods recommended more often could be placed at the bottom with less frequent ones toward to top. Though the Swedish board chose not to use the pyramid, the food retailer did. And ever since, the pyramid has become a popular visual aid to explain dietary strategies.

Since that time, a number of diet pyramids have been designed. The USDA used a food pyramid from 1992 until 2011 before "MyPlate" finally replaced nearly two decades of a healthy food pyramid promotion. Other dietary pyramids have been designed around cultural foods and diets, such as those describing foods associated with Asian and African heritage. Others provide a diagram to better understand how often specific foods should be eaten within a diet plan. All you need to do is glance at the pyramid and quickly appreciate which foods should be eaten daily, weekly or monthly. This makes planning your meals within any diet that much easier.

FASTING
DAYS

PARTIAL FASTING
DAYS/TRANSITION
DAYS

NON-FASTING DAYS

While the Intermittent Fasting Pyramid does not necessarily tell you exactly which foods to eat and how often, it does provide the same basic visual principles to help you adopt an intermittent fasting diet. With the Intermittent Fasting Pyramid, you will be able to eat your regular diet most days. These days will be represented on the bottom of the pyramid. During your fasting day, you will have reduced caloric intake. Your fasting day only occurs once each week and will be located at the top of the pyramid. And days in the middle of the pyramid will reflect a transition period between your regular diet and your fasting diet. Given this, you can appreciate why a pyramid is an ideal structure for providing a diagrammatic representation of this unique intermittent fasting approach.

## The Intermittent Fasting Diet Explained

At this point, you probably appreciate all the potential health and weight loss benefits intermittent fasting offers. But despite these advantages, and even with modified fasting plans that allow reduced caloric intake, it can still be difficult to stick to your diet. While the rationale behind the Intermittent Fasting Pyramid will be explained in greater detail in the next chapter, suffice it to say that the pyramid approach enhances your chances of success for losing weight and in achieving wellness by making your intermittent fasting diet more enjoyable.

In essence, the Intermittent Fasting Pyramid offers three levels or tiers that represent the different days of the week. For the sake of simplicity, Day 1 can represent Monday each week. Because this fasting day is only a single day each week, it is located at the top of the pyramid. Day 2 and Day 3, Tuesday and Wednesday, are considered transition days. During transition days, you do not eat as much as you normally would, but you do eat more than you did when fasting. Transition days are located in the middle level of the Intermittent Fasting Pyramid. Lastly, Day 4, Day 5, Day 6, and Day 7, which represent the rest of the week, are days where you eat a healthy diet with a normal number of calories. Because these are the most frequent days of the diet, these are located at the base of the Intermittent Fasting Pyramid.

Notably, the number of calories you are allowed to eat during your fasting day and transition days will vary based on your gender, age, height, and level of activity. For example, women require fewer calories in most instances when compared to men. Likewise, as we age, our metabolism slows requiring fewer calories as well. A typical range for a fasting day may therefore vary between 500 and 800 calories while transition days are commonly between 1000 and 1200 calories. Calculating these precise determinations will be further described later in the book. Regardless, these figures provide a rough estimate for you in determining the calorie restriction you will need.

## Great for Weight Loss, Great for Health, Great for Everyone!

The Intermittent Fasting Pyramid is a program that promotes both weight loss and better health, especially when choosing predominantly healthy foods within your meal plans. At the same time, it is a much more tolerable way to enjoy the benefits of fasting without experiencing some of the common pitfalls associated with it. For one, you will experience less hunger than you would with complete fasting as you are allowed 25 percent of your normal calories during your intermittent fasting day. And during transition days, you are allowed 50 percent of your normal calories. This intermittent fasting plan makes fasting more easily tolerated while preserving all the advantages of intermittent fasting!

In addition, the Intermittent Fasting Pyramid is great for individuals who want to lose weight quickly. But it can also be modified for those who simply want to maintain a healthy weight or even intermittently shed just a few pounds. Given its inherent flexibility, the Intermittent Fasting Pyramid can be used in different ways. For example, if you are looking to only shed a few pounds or to maintain your healthy weight, you may choose to be less restrictive on your fasting day and your transition days. However, the pyramid as outlined will result in rapid weight loss. Should you want to slow your weight loss, you can simply increase your calories on your fasting and partial fasting days. Or, you can choose to include only one partial fasting day rather than two. The Intermittent Fasting Pyramid naturally offers a degree of flexibility as long as you stay within the scope of the pyramid structure. Regardless whether you are seeking steady weight loss over time, periodic weight loss when needed, or simply better health in general, the Intermittent Fasting Pyramid provides a great strategy to achieve your goals.

# CHAPTER 5:

# Why the Pyramid Works

Each year, experts and panels rank various dieting programs based on the benefits they provide for weight loss and health. In fact, more than three-dozen diets are routinely evaluated each year to determine how effective they are in facilitating health and wellness. Depending on which review you read, different rankings and opinions may result, which can make it challenging to know which diet is actually the best. Regardless, it remains important to assess whether a diet can achieve the goals you want based on expert analysis and dieting experiences.

When it comes to fasting and intermittent fasting programs, plenty of research supports its effectiveness in achieving both weight loss and improved health. As far as weight loss, fasting results in reduced insulin levels and less insulin resistance at a cellular level. This means cells use glucose more efficiently, which improves metabolism. At the same time, fasting inherently boosts your metabolism and encourages the liver to turn body fat into sugars to be used for energy. These key fasting effects thus serve to rid your body of stored fat and help you slim down.[10]

In addition to weight loss, fasting also lowers your heart rate and blood pressure, allows better stress tolerance, and reduces the amount of inflammation in your body. These effects have advantages for aging and longevity as well as for your quality of life.[11] Certainly, weight loss and health benefits of fasting and intermittent fasting have been recognized, but the important question is how best to introduce intermittent fasting into your life. You may be well convinced that intermittent fasting is a great way to meet your goals. But what is the best approach to pursue an intermittent fasting diet?

Different intermittent fasting programs exist, but when it comes to one that greatly improves your chances of success, the Intermittent Fasting Pyramid is the best. While dieting pyramids certainly offer a visual guide to help you approach a dieting plan, the Intermittent Fasting Pyramid is a very effective health and weight loss strategy for many other reasons. In fact, it reduces many of the challenges that other intermittent fasting programs pose while still offering the same great results. This is a major reason why people are embracing the Intermittent Fasting Pyramid as their preferred method of intermittent fasting. And once you appreciate the advantages it provides, you will likely choose to incorporate the Intermittent Fasting Pyramid into your life.

## Common Challenges Associated with Intermittent Fasting

Before describing why the Intermittent Fasting Pyramid is so effective, some of the difficulties that people often experience with intermittent fasting should be identified. In doing so, you will better appreciate the advantages that the Intermittent Fasting Pyramid offers. Understanding this, you can likely guess the most frequent complaint associated with intermittent fasting…hunger! If you have ever performed a complete fast, then you know that going without food for many hours or days can be pretty unpleasant. Even if you're required to only reduce your caloric intake, hunger pains can still be an issue.

Of course, hunger is not unique to intermittent fasting. Most diets restrict the total number of calories consumed, and therefore, hunger is often a part of most dieting programs. But the intensity and degree of hunger you experience matters. With fasting, and to a lesser extent with intermittent fasting, the hunger can be more intense during your fasting days. And though weight loss may provide positive feedback to help you stick to the diet plan, hunger can undermine your best intentions. Thus, while immediate discomfort is one issue, the inability to stay the course with intermittent fasting due to hunger is a larger concern.

While hunger is not unique to intermittent fasting, other challenges are. Specifically, one of the most significant problems associated with intermittent fasting involves binge-eating after a fast has been completed. One of the most popular intermittent fasting programs is the 5:2 program where reduced caloric intake is required for two days each week and normal eating patterns are allowed for the other five days. While the reduced number of calories consumed during the fasting days offers weight loss and health benefits, overeating immediately after a fasting day can undermine your weight loss goals. In other words, a common challenge for many on intermittent fasting diets is trying to avoid this yo-yo pattern of fasting and binging.

Lastly, one additional complaint with intermittent fasting is its potential to interfere with other life activities. Of course, any dietary restrictions may make it challenging to dine at a restaurant while adhering to a meal plan. Likewise, avoiding certain foods and beverages can be difficult with any diet that limits food types or calories. But the episodic nature of intermittent fasting can make these challenges more pronounced. This is especially true when fasting days fall on a weekend or during some festive occasion where additional pressures to abort your fast are present.

Despite all the advantages that intermittent fasting can provide, these aspects of most intermittent fasting plans can be problematic. Hunger, binging, and general frustrations can convince you that sticking to the diet just isn't worth it. But nothing could be farther from the truth. The solution is not to give up your plans for intermittent fasting altogether but to approach intermittent fasting from a new perspective. And that is where the Intermittent Fasting Pyramid offers its unique advantages.

## A Better Way to Intermittently Fast

With the Intermittent Fasting Pyramid, you will be more likely to stick to an intermittent fasting plan, and in addition, you will have a more pleasant experience along the way. At the same time, the Intermittent Fasting Pyramid helps you to better realize the advantages that intermittent fasting can offer in terms of both weight loss and better health. The following are the major reasons why the Intermittent Fasting Pyramid is a better way to approach intermittent fasting regardless of the primary goals you have in mind.

- **Reduces the Intensity of Hunger** – As you recall, the Intermittent Fasting Pyramid is a modified intermittent fasting program that only requires a reduction in calories rather than a complete fast. Specifically, the amount allowed during your fasting day is 25 percent of your normal caloric requirements based on age, height, gender, and activity levels. But rather than having this restriction imposed 2 or more days each week, the Intermittent Fasting Pyramid only requires this degree of calorie restriction for a single day. Then, during transition days, you can have 50 percent of your normal caloric requirements. The end result is that you will experience less hunger each week and be much more likely to stay on track with your diet. And that means you will also see better results over time!

- **Extends the Fasting Process (and Benefits!)** – As described, the transition days in the Intermittent Fasting Pyramid allow you to gradually return to your normal caloric intake. However, these transition days have other benefits as well. For one, transition days extend the fasting process during the week through continued caloric restriction. This allows you to continue to enjoy the weight loss advantages of intermittent fasting for a total of 3 days each week, which exceeds common intermittent fasting diets that only include 2 days of fasting. In addition, the extension of calorie restriction during the transition days might also boost other health benefits. Thus, transition days offer an approach that better optimizes the advantages of intermittent fasting by encouraging you to fast more days in a less intense manner.

- **Decreases the Risk of Post-Fast Binges** – A major issue that has been associated with intermittent fasting is binge-eating immediately after a day of fasting. Having struggled through the fast, it's natural to want to compensate on your next regular day of eating. But this undermines the advantages of intermittent fasting in terms of both weight loss and health promotion. The Intermittent Fasting Pyramid, however, reduces this risk by allowing 2 transition days to follow your fasting day. During these transition days, you must still adhere to a degree of calorie restriction, but the restrictions are not as severe. As a result, you are able to ease back into your normal diet, and the urge to binge is less. Ultimately, this leads to better results and greater confidence that you will succeed in attaining your goals.

- **Lets You Live Your Life** – In examining the structure of the Intermittent Fasting Pyramid, the bottom level of the pyramid allows you to have a total of 4 days each week to eat regularly. If you align these 4 days with the end of the week, the impact fasting may have on your lifestyle will be remarkably less. Many choose to fast on Monday, transition on Tuesday and Wednesday, and then have the rest of the week to enjoy meals without excessive restrictions. This approach allows your dieting plan to interfere as little as possible with social events and other activities. Likewise, you can structure the days of your Intermittent Fasting Pyramid however you like so that it aligns best with your weekly schedule. This is yet another reason why the Intermittent Fasting Pyramid is being increasingly adopted as a dietary strategy.

## A Logical Approach Backed by Science

As you can appreciate, the Intermittent Fasting Pyramid addresses many of the major challenges associated with intermittent fasting diets. Limiting intense fasting times while adding transitional days offers a common sense approach to intermittent fasting. And at the same time, it increases your chances of success because you tolerate the calorie restrictions much better. But these advantages are not the only reasons the Intermittent Fasting Pyramid is so attractive. Science has shown a number of weight loss and health benefits associated with intermittent fasting in general that also support use of the Intermittent Fasting Pyramid.

In the next chapters, the facts supporting intermittent fasting as a weight loss and wellness approach will be highlighted. Over the course of the last few decades, significant research has been conducted demonstrating that the advantages of intermittent fasting are indeed real. Understanding these revelations will further help you appreciate why this dieting strategy has so much potential. And combining this knowledge with the Intermittent Fasting Pyramid structure will allow you to reap these benefits in your own life.

SECTION III:

# The Facts

# CHAPTER 6:

# What Science and Research is Telling Us About Intermittent Fasting

Since 2012, a number of authors, advocates, and even celebrities have emerged supporting the use of intermittent fasting diets. The use of intermittent fasting as a weight loss technique has thus become increasingly popular. But you may not realize many other advantages are now being recognized between intermittent fasting and overall health. Is all this hype actually supported by research and science? Or are these claims simply anecdotal in nature reflecting the experience of a few individuals who have tried intermittent fasting?

In the past, research concerning intermittent fasting mainly involved animal studies. Experiments using mice and monkeys had been the primary data available by which the effects of intermittent fasting were examined. While these studies showed promising results, there was a major problem...they weren't human studies. Therefore, solid proof that intermittent fasting was actually beneficial for weight loss and other health problems for us was still lacking. Fortunately, that is no longer the case, as each year several new studies involving intermittent fasting are being published.

In this chapter, we will discuss the current state of science as it pertains to intermittent fasting. While other chapters will go into greater detail about the health effects and weight loss associated with intermittent fasting, an overview of current research will be provided supporting the use of intermittent fasting for a number of health reasons. And recent insights about how intermittent fasting provides these health advantages will also be discussed. As a result, you will have a much better appreciation for how intermittent fasting provides for better health and wellness.

## A Snapshot of Intermittent Fasting Research Today

When looking at the available research concerning intermittent fasting, a few things become pretty apparent. First, much of the research before this century was conducted on animals. For whatever reason, a desire to study fasting among human subjects didn't seem to be present. But even so, studies of mice and other laboratory animals were showing positive effects when diets were restricted. Eventually, this led to a greater interest and investigations in looking at the effects of fasting in human populations. Thankfully, this is now resulting in an increasing number of research studies.

Early research studies related to the effects of fasting in human populations involved fairly small numbers of participants. This limited the ability to make clear conclusions about the effects of intermittent fasting. At the same time, the studies tended to use different types of intermittent fasting diets, which made it harder to compare results as well. Also, many of these experiments didn't measure the same things each time. While nearly all looked at weight loss, some looked at glucose and insulin levels while others assessed changes in cholesterol values.[12] Though a sense that intermittent fasting was beneficial was growing, clear determinations about its effects on health and wellness were not yet available.

In the last few years, however, things have changed. Summary reviews of several research studies are now available that critiques their findings and provides insights about intermittent fasting effects.[13] Of course, much research still needs to be performed in order to gain greater clarity about its effects on weight loss and health, but things are certainly better than they were. In addition to many research studies on intermittent fasting showing weight loss advantages, the majority also show positive effects on metabolism, inflammation, and lipid control. And a fair number are showing benefits in mood and cognition from intermittent fasting as well. In other words, science is finally showing support for intermittent fasting to match what millions have been practicing for centuries.

Another important insight about today's available research on intermittent fasting involves the types of diets that have been studied. In various reviews, intermittent fasting diet types are distinguished based on the intensity and duration of the fasts used.[14] For example, some intermittent fasting diets use complete all-day fasts where no food is consumed for 24 hours. These are the more traditional fasts that have been associated with religious fasting over centuries. However, most intermittent fasting diets are not this restrictive today.

Other types of intermittent fasting diets require only a reduction in calories during fasting days. Naturally, these are not as restrictive or as intense. These are termed modified fasting regimens with an allowance of 20-25 percent of your normal calories typically being permitted during these fasting days.[15] And still other intermittent fasting diets in research studies are labeled time-restricted fasting diets. These diet types only allow eating to occur during certain hours of each day.[16] As you can appreciate, each of these intermittent fasting diet types might have different effects on both weight and health.

With this in mind, the majority of the research that has been conducted involves modified fasting regimens where partial calorie restriction occurs on fasting days. An example of this type of diet would be the 5:2 intermittent fasting diet, where 2 days each week allow only 25 percent of your normal calories to be consumed. More than a dozen studies have now explored this type of intermittent fasting approach, and thus, it has the most research evidence behind it. Likewise, these studies have also explored how intermittent fasting diets might actually work in improving our overall health.[17]

## Research Theories About Intermittent Fasting

When it comes to intermittent fasting, certainly a reduction in the calories you eat might explain why weight loss could occur. But intermittent fasting is different from regular diets in this area. Other diets restrict calories continuously either by focusing on different food types (quality) or by limiting the amount of food you eat (quantity). In contrast, intermittent fasting typically permits a relatively normal diet in between fasting times. Though higher quality of food chosen is typically encouraged, one may well consume the same number of calories over time as they normally would.

Understanding this, the mechanism by which intermittent

fasting causes weight loss has been a focus of some investigations. In addition, intermittent fasting offers a number of other health benefits besides weight loss, which will be described in greater detail later. Because of this, research studies have offered theories about intermittent fasting and how it provides the health benefits it does. Based on several observations, three main scientific theories exist in this regard. These theories involve our bodies' daily circadian rhythm, our gastrointestinal tract, and associated lifestyle changes we may make while fasting.[18]

The first theory has the most amount of support when it comes to scientific study. As you may be aware, our circadian rhythm refers to the daily fluctuations that our bodies experience on a regular basis. Sleep patterns, the speed of our metabolism, and the production of different hormones fluctuate throughout the day. Jet lag is a perfect example of how we can be negatively affected when we are out of sync with our circadian cycles. For each of us, the timing of when we eat can therefore affect various aspects of our health. This occurs because our bodies change throughout the day based on our circadian rhythm patterns.[19]

With this in mind, it has been shown that fasting during certain times of the day are better than others. For instance, early in the day, our bodies handle calories more easily, our metabolism is faster, and our stomach digests foods more quickly. In contrast, the opposite occurs in the evening. Thus, one theory supports that fasting in the evening hours offers weight loss and health benefits because it better aligns with the body's natural rhythms. And in fact, eating meals at times that are not well-aligned to our circadian rhythms have been linked to higher rates of obesity, diabetes, heart disease and breast cancer.[20]

While intermittent fasting may exert some weight and health

benefits by being in sync with our circadian rhythm, another theory suggests intermittent fasting has beneficial effects on our digestive system.[21] Throughout our intestinal tract, millions of microorganisms exist that actually influence not only our digestion but our health as well. These organisms have been collectively called our "microbiome," and together, they can either exert a positive influence on our health or a negative one. Research exploring our microbiome and how it affects health is a hot area of investigation today.

While many things can affect the types of microorganisms we have in our microbiome, our diet is a major one. Because of this, one theory suggests that intermittent fasting improves health by positively influencing the various bacteria lining our intestinal tract. Going back to evolutionary considerations, it has been suggested that intermittent fasting mimics the way human beings ate throughout time. Therefore, reverting back to this type of diet might invite a microbiome that enhances health and wellness. Though much research is needed in this field, the theory provides a logical consideration in describing how intermittent fasting might exert its positive effects.

Lastly, some research has suggested that intermittent fasting invites other lifestyle changes that might improve health concurrently. For example, choosing to intermittently fast might change the type of foods you eat, which might lead to better health and weight loss. Fasting might improve sleep, which could boost metabolism while giving you more energy for calorie-burning activities. And intermittent fasting has been shown to improve mood and self-confidence, which could encourage exercise and healthier behaviors. Though not as potentially robust as the other theories concerning intermittent fasting, lifestyle changes might also be a mechanism explaining why intermittent fasting offers health advantages.

## The Bottom Line Regarding Intermittent Fasting

In the next chapter, the specific health advantages that intermittent fasting provides will be described in greater detail. But as an overview, research is progressively showing that intermittent fasting offers an array of health benefits. By far, the majority show that intermittent fasting provides clear advantages in weight loss and achieving a healthy weight. At the same time, research demonstrates that intermittent fasting frequently lowers cholesterol levels, reduces inflammation in the body, and boosts metabolism. These effects have widespread implications including the tendency for intermittent fasting to lower risks for heart disease, diabetes and cancer.

Based on these findings, it is clear that intermittent fasting offers more than just a weight loss diet. It also provides a means to improve your overall health and wellness while achieving the weight loss goals you want. And because intermittent fasting does not require constant calorie reductions, it is often better tolerated with less hunger and frustration. This is especially true for modified fasting diets that only require a reduction in the calories consumed on fasting days. All of these aspects of intermittent fasting are now supported by science, and because of this, the incentive to consider intermittent fasting as a dietary lifestyle is that much greater.

# CHAPTER 7:

# Health Benefits Beyond Weight Loss with Intermittent Fasting

The health benefits of intermittent fasting, other than weight loss, have been well appreciated for centuries. In fact, fasting itself was not intended to be a practice to lose weight but instead promote spiritual and physical wellbeing. Its use for weight management and weight loss has been a more recent trend. Therefore, it stands to reason that you should know the facts supporting the use of intermittent fasting in promoting overall wellness. In many ways, these benefits are even more substantial than those associated with weight loss. In other words, you get more bang for your buck!

It is also worth noting that science has come a long way in identifying these additional health benefits linked to intermittent fasting. For example, research now shows how intermittent fasting can improve your metabolism, reduce the amount of inflammation in your body, and even slow down aging. While some of these benefits might be attributed to better weight management, intermittent fasting directly provides these health advantages as well. The following describes what research has shown thus far in relation to these other intermittent fasting benefits.

## Intermittent Fasting and Your Heart

When it comes to heart disease, intermittent fasting provides health advantages in a few different ways. First, studies have shown that intermittent fasting can lower levels of cholesterol and triglycerides. One study involving 20 individuals who were obese showed that an intermittent fasting diet for 8 weeks significantly lowered their lipid levels. And among all research studies involving intermittent fasting, more than a third that assessed cholesterol effects showed significant improvements.[22] Given the link between high cholesterol and the risk for heart disease, these findings show how intermittent fasting can lower your heart disease risk.

In addition to lowering your lipid levels, intermittent fasting also reduces heart disease risk in other ways. Studies have shown that intermittent fasting can be associated with fewer inflammatory markers in the body. Specifically, one researcher showed that intermittent fasting lowered an inflammatory protein called C-Reactive protein after 12 weeks. And reviews of several research studies have also noted that 40 percent of relevant studies evaluating intermittent fasting showed lowered levels of inflammation in the body.[23] Because inflammation is linked to atherosclerosis, blood vessel damage, and high blood pressure, this is another way that intermittent fasting promotes better heart health.

## Intermittent Fasting and Diabetes

It's no secret that a number of people with diabetes are either overweight or obese. In fact, excess weight is a risk factor for developing Type II diabetes. As we gain excess weight, increasing demands are placed on our metabolism to properly manage blood glucose and insulin levels. As diabetes begins to develop, cells become increasingly resistant to insulin, which causes rises in blood sugar. And at the same time, the pancreas tries to pump out more insulin to overcome the cell resistance to insulin. This explains why researchers not only look at glucose levels but insulin levels as well when assessing diabetic risks.

With this in mind, several studies have examined whether or not intermittent fasting reduces the risk for developing diabetes. The most significant study in this regard involved 107 diabetic women who were placed on an intermittent fasting diet for 6 months. Despite weight loss not being significant, they showed a significant drop in their insulin levels. In addition, they also showed improvements in their bodies' abilities to respond to insulin overall. This is not an isolated finding. In fact, 40 percent of research studies examining insulin levels and intermittent fasting showed a reduction with diabetic risk.[24] Thus, while weight loss does lower the risk for diabetes and/or enhance its management, intermittent fasting provides additional benefits in these areas unrelated to the weight loss it provides.

## Intermittent Fasting and Cancer

While no direct studies regarding cancer occurrence among individuals who intermittently fast have been conducted to date, indirect studies suggest that intermittent fasting is beneficial here as well. Research does exist that has looked at molecules in the blood linked to higher cancer risk. For instance, one study involving 30 subjects showed a reduction in leptin levels among intermittent fasting participants. Leptin is an inflammatory marker sometimes associated with breast cancer.[25] In another study involving 10 people, specific tumor factors were significantly lowered during intermittent fasting.[26] Though not definitive, this would suggest intermittent fasting does reduce overall cancer risk.

In considering how intermittent fasting might reduce cancer risk, one theory suggests that reduced levels of body inflammation might be important. Just as increased inflammation can cause a higher risk of heart disease, inflammation also increases the chance for developing various types of cancer. Understanding this, intermittent fasting may reduce inflammation in a number of ways. For one, fasting could result in a healthier intestinal microbiome that reduces inflammation in the body. Similarly, more efficient metabolism and immune system function may occur with intermittent fasting, which could also reduce inflammation.[27] While additional research is needed to clarify these issues, everything so far supports a lower cancer risk when you choose an intermittent fasting diet.

## Intermittent Fasting and Your Brain

When it comes to fasting in general, research has shown that many people struggle with the associated hunger that may develop. In fact, some studies have shown that the hunger associated with fasting may persist over time without any significant improvement.[28] Naturally, this would negatively affect the ability to stick to a diet. But when you examine fasting practices in greater detail, this research is actually describing complete all-day fasts that require complete calorie restriction. When it comes to modified fasting practices requiring reductions in calorie intake on fasting days only, hunger issues are dramatically less.

In research evaluating modified types of intermittent fasting, less than 15 percent of people describe being hungry, frustrated, or irritable. Similarly, other common symptoms associated with fasting, like low levels of energy and being cold, are also infrequent with modified fasting protocols. In fact, in most cases, intermittent fasting is associated with improved mood and higher levels of self-confidence. Surveys have also shown that perceived stress levels, mood swings, and overall fatigue actually improve with intermittent fasting.[29] These reflect important benefits that other diets cannot necessarily claim.

Lastly, intermittent fasting has been associated with improved attention, concentration and memory. Interestingly enough, these benefits were appreciated by the ancient Egyptians who required fasting for some students before they began their academic studies. And most of us are familiar with the phenomenon of a "food coma" after eating a large meal, especially after that turkey at Thanksgiving! Though the precise mechanisms by which intermittent fasting enhances clarity of thought are not well-defined, some researchers suggest intermittent fasting might alter the brain's neurotransmitters in a favorable way. Perhaps this also helps explain why religions have encouraged fasting throughout time as a way to enhance meditative practices.

## More Than Just a Weight Loss Approach

Understandably, most people primarily consider intermittent fasting as a way to lose weight. Several books encourage different types of fasting plans as a dieting technique, and indeed, intermittent fasting is very effective in this regard. But at the same time, it offers so much more in terms of overall wellness. From digestion, to metabolic effects, to reducing the risk of a number of health conditions, intermittent fasting promotes better health in several ways. And research is progressively showing the benefits that intermittent fasting can provide.

Certainly, much more has yet to be discovered about the mechanisms and the advantages that intermittent fasting offers. However, much more is known today than was known a decade ago. This accounts in part for its increasing popularity as a dietary choice and as a weight loss strategy. As additional research reveals new insights about intermittent fasting, however, support for its use will likely grow. But even now, more than enough research shows why choosing intermittent fasting can be a great decision.

# CHAPTER 8:

# Weight Loss – What to Expect

Most of us who have tried multiple diets over the years appreciate that not all diets offer the same degree of weight loss. Some can help you shed some pounds quickly while others are more gradual in their effects. Likewise, some diets are meant to be more of a longstanding lifestyle change while others offer a temporary way to reach a weight loss target. When it comes to intermittent fasting, however, this type of diet can be used for both purposes. Thus, the type of intermittent fasting diet you choose should align with your own personal weight loss goals.

The Intermittent Fasting Pyramid adopts an approach that encourages modified fasting during your fasting day and your transition days. The term modified simply implies that during these days, your fast will require a reduction in calories rather than a complete avoidance of all foods. For your fasting day, you should consume 25 percent of your normal calories while transition days allow half your normal caloric intake. Using these recommendations as a guide, weight loss with the Intermittent Fasting Pyramid can be estimated fairly accurately. Because research has actually examined the average weight loss with this type of intermittent fasting approach, average weight loss expected with this diet can be estimated.

The recommended calorie restriction with the Intermittent

Fasting Pyramid allows for a modified approach to fasting. As a result, it may be considered more of a lifestyle diet that helps maintain weight loss over time. Although the fasting day and partial fasting day caloric intake is defined in detail, options to tailor the Intermittent Fasting Pyramid to meet your own specific weight loss goals also exist. These options will be covered later in the book allowing you to customize your own personal intermittent fasting program. But for now, this chapter will provide information about the weight you can expect to lose using the Intermittent Fasting Pyramid in its standard form.

## Intermittent Fasting and Weight Loss Mechanisms

The Intermittent Fasting Pyramid has been shown to help people lose weight while also improving overall health and longevity. But exactly how does this diet program actually result in weight loss? Interestingly, there are more than one mechanism by which intermittent fasting helps you lose weight. While most diets help you lose weight by restricting the number of calories you can have every day, intermittent fasting promotes weight loss in three different ways. This is one reason why the Intermittent Fasting Pyramid helps you better realize your weight loss goals.

The first way intermittent fasting promotes weight loss is by reducing the amount food (and calories) consumed each week. Naturally, when you restrict the number of calories you eat during your fasting and transition days, you will lose weight week after week as long as you don't overcompensate during your regular eating days. In this way, intermittent fasting has been shown to be comparable to other diets that simply reduce dietary food calories continuously.[30] But unlike these other diets, intermittent fasting lets you have a break several days each week where you may eat normally. This makes intermittent fasting better tolerated as a result by comparison.

While calorie reduction is important for weight loss, intermittent fasting boosts your overall metabolism. Through hormonal changes and effects on the insulin and glucose system, your body is able to burn calories better when you intermittently fast. This means that not only will you have fewer calories being consumed, but at the same time, your body will be burning calories at a higher rate.[31] This is the second way in which intermittent fasting helps promote weight loss.

Lastly, intermittent fasting targets specific areas where you will lose your weight. Notably, intermittent fasting increases your body's metabolism of fat. That means the weight you lose will be more likely to come from fatty tissues than from other areas. When you fast, your body's metabolism shifts gears and starts using fats for energy instead of glucose. This has important implications not only in your ability to lose weight but also in losing the weight where you would like.[32] This also makes intermittent fasting a very attractive diet program compared to other conventional diets.

## Intermittent Fasting and Average Weight Loss Results

Several studies have been conducted that examined the amount of weight people have lost while on intermittent fasting diets. The majority of these studies have compared intermittent fasting with other diets that restrict caloric intake continuously.

Interestingly, the research shows that intermittent fasting offers the same amount of weight loss as these other diets in terms of total pounds lost. In essence, over 1 to 3 months, you should expect to lose between 4 to 8 percent of your body weight using an intermittent fasting plan like the one outlined in the Intermittent Fasting Pyramid.[33]

What does this mean in real terms? Let's suppose you weigh 140 pounds when you decide to start using the Intermittent Fasting Pyramid. The potential weight loss you can expect to lose over a couple of months would be somewhere between 5.5 to 11 pounds. This is supported by other research that found people tend to lose just over half of a pound each week when using an intermittent fasting diet.[34] This figure is the same amount of weight loss you would expect to lose on average with other diets. Thus, this shows that intermittent fasting is at least as effective for weight loss as other dieting options long-term.

The advantages of the Intermittent Fasting Pyramid in terms of better tolerance, less frustrations, and other health benefits make this dietary approach more attractive than other diets when you realize the potential for weight loss is the same. But intermittent fasting has additional weight loss benefits besides just the total number of pounds you can expect to lose. Intermittent fasting also results in greater amounts of fatty tissue being lost while preserving your lean muscle mass. While about 25 percent of the weight lost in other diets can be attributed to reduced muscle mass, only 10 percent of the weight lost with intermittent fasting is from muscle.[35] Therefore, not only does intermittent fasting allow you to lose the same amount of weight by comparison, but it also helps you lose excess fatty tissue to a greater degree.

## Intermittent Fasting Pyramid – Have Your Weight Loss and Health Too!

Given the evidence described, intermittent fasting offers a steady and effective diet strategy that helps you lose weight. In addition to losing the same amount of weight as with other diets, intermittent fasting allows you to lose weight where you want. On average, people who choose intermittent fasting see their waistlines shrink as much as 7 percent over a few weeks. And for many, the intermittent nature of this dietary program is much preferred and better tolerated when compared to other diet options.

The weight loss that you can expect using the Intermittent Fasting Pyramid is significant. Also, intermittent fasting enhances your health and longevity through a number of mechanisms already described. And at the same time, you can choose to be more aggressive in the caloric restriction during your fasting and transition days to potentially increase the weight loss effect. In any case, you can rest assured the Intermittent Fasting Pyramid can help you achieve your weight loss goals while also improving your overall wellness.

SECTION IV:

# Do's and Don'ts

# CHAPTER 9:

# Who Should do Intermittent Fasting?

As previously discussed, the Intermittent Fasting Pyramid offers a number of health advantages. These include the chance to better realize the weight loss you want in addition to many other benefits involving your metabolism, your heart health, and your longevity. Therefore, intermittent fasting has been increasingly recognized as a great way to reach specific weight loss and wellness goals. Because intermittent fasting offers comparable weight loss to other types of diets, the additional health "perks" makes intermittent fasting diets quite attractive. And the Intermittent Fasting Pyramid further enhances this attractiveness by making intermittent fasting less frustrating and more enjoyable.

Given the popularity of intermittent fasting, many people are interested in choosing the Intermittent Fasting Pyramid. But, who is the Intermittent Fasting Pyramid for?

## The Intermittent Fasting Pyramid – A Weight Loss Remedy for Past Failures

When it comes to dieting, many of us realize that our dieting efforts often fall short of our expectations. Even with the strongest of commitments, setbacks and unexpected obstacles can interfere with our dieting success regardless of the diet selected.

Likewise, not every dietary approach works for everyone, which means you might need to cycle through a few before finding one that works best for you. Understanding these challenges, the Intermittent Fasting Pyramid is designed to minimize these frustrations and increase the chance that your dieting efforts will be successful. That doesn't mean that it is guaranteed to work for everybody, but its unique approach to intermittent fasting does improve the odds tremendously.

The Intermittent Fasting Pyramid is something that should be considered by anyone who has struggled with other diets. In fact, even if you have had problems sticking to an intermittent fasting diet in the past, the Intermittent Fasting Pyramid might be your solution. Common struggles with intermittent fasting include an inability to tolerate the hunger on fasting days as well as binge-eating after the fast is over. If these were challenges for you previously when trying intermittent fasting, then the Intermittent Fasting Pyramid may be much better tolerated, which will naturally improve your chances of achieving your goals.

It should also be noted that the Intermittent Fasting Pyramid can boost the results of other diets, especially if you have "stalled out" in your weight loss efforts. A few options exist here. For one, you may choose to simply switch to the Intermittent Fasting Pyramid for a few weeks before resuming your regular dieting plan. Or, alternatively, you may combine your current diet program with the Intermittent Fasting Pyramid. In other words, you adopt the Intermittent Fasting Pyramid structure, but you follow your specific diet. For example, lets say you are on a keto diet but your weight loss has stalled. You can combine your keto diet with the Intermittent Fasting Pyramid structure.

This new approach will likely kick-start your weight loss. Both of these techniques may give your weight loss efforts a boost and help you attain your overall goals.

## The Intermittent Fasting Pyramid – An Option for Targeted Body Sculpting

One major advantage of intermittent fasting is its ability to promote weight loss in areas that are primarily "fatty" in nature. In contrast to other diets, intermittent fasting tends to preserve lean muscle mass while specifically targeting fatty tissue. As a result, you lose weight in areas that are often the most problematic without sacrificing a muscular physique. Thus, for those wanting to "sculpt" their body in a specific way, the Intermittent Fasting Pyramid is an attractive dietary approach.

The way that intermittent fasting achieves this body sculpting effect is through intermittent ketosis. During fasting periods, less glucose is available in the diet due to calorie restriction. As a result, the liver "switches gears" and starts to break down fats instead of sugars, which is how ketosis occurs. During this time, fats in the body become the primary targets for weight loss. Once fasting is over, however, normal sugar metabolism resumes.[36] It appears this back-and-forth nature of ketosis and regular glucose metabolism typical of intermittent fasting diets is what selectively targets fatty tissue for weight loss while preserving muscle.

With this in mind, the Intermittent Fasting Pyramid can be a great choice if you are having trouble eliminating weight in certain problem areas of your body. Excess belly fat, fatty tissue in the inner thighs and buttocks, and other common areas where adipose tissue is deposited may respond quite well to this intermittent fasting strategy. If other diets have failed in this regard, the Intermittent Fasting Pyramid is certainly worth a try.

## The Intermittent Fasting Pyramid – A Plan for Overall Health and Wellness

Most people have heard of intermittent fasting as a weight loss plan even if they haven't yet tried it. But as described, intermittent fasting offers many other health advantages beyond weight loss. In fact, the popularity of the intermittent fasting diet grew after Michael Mosley showcased the diet's capacity to improve glucose metabolism and reduce diabetic risk.[37] With this in mind, many people who have specific health issues may benefit from trying the Intermittent Fasting Pyramid.

Some individuals with specific health conditions may want to consider intermittent fasting as a diet strategy. Individuals with hypertension might benefit from intermittent fasting since it has been shown to be effective in reducing blood pressure levels. Likewise, individuals with poor concentration and attention may also benefit from intermittent fasting. And anyone who wishes to slow down the aging process might want to consider intermittent fasting. In each of these instances, the Intermittent Fasting Pyramid can offer better health and wellbeing.

While many health benefits have been associated with intermittent fasting, as mentioned previously, individuals with diabetes in particular might consider intermittent fasting as a diet and weight loss plan. Fasting improves your body's cellular response to insulin, which in turn, improves the metabolism of glucose. By allowing your body's cells to intermittently go without constant glucose stimulation, fasting gives them a chance to become more responsive to your natural insulin levels. Ultimately, this not only promotes weight loss but may also reduce your need for medications. If you have diabetes, you may want to consider intermittent fasting, but be sure to check with your physician about any specific precautions that might need to be taken.

## Is the Intermittent Fasting Pyramid Right for You?

Intermittent fasting isn't simply a diet plan for people wanting to lose weight. Intermittent fasting can be a great diet program for a number of health problems as well. Individuals who have struggled with other diets, including some intermittent fasting plans, can potentially benefit from the Intermittent Fasting Pyramid. So can others with specific health conditions. This makes it an attractive option that some will want to seriously consider in pursuing your weight loss and health goals.

While the Intermittent Fasting Pyramid can help many achieve the weight loss and health they want, there are some people who should avoid intermittent fasting as a choice. In the next chapter, we will discuss situations where intermittent fasting might need to be avoided or may require some additional precautions. However, the vast majority of people can truly benefit from the Intermittent Fasting Pyramid in their pursuit of better weight management and enhanced overall wellness. However, as with any change in diet and especially with any diet that involves calorie restriction, it is important to check with your doctor before starting the program.

# CHAPTER 10:

# Who Should avoid Intermittent Fasting?

Several weight loss diets are available that might offer you specific benefits and advantages. However, not everyone will respond to a particular diet in the same way as each of us are unique, and this pertains to intermittent fasting as well. Understanding this, intermittent fasting as well as the Intermittent Fasting Pyramid may not be for everyone as some people might not tolerate the meal scheduling or they may simply prefer other options. It is noteworthy, however, that some people should avoid intermittent fasting altogether because of the inherent nature of the diet itself. In this chapter, we will discuss specific conditions and groups of people for whom intermittent fasting may not be the ideal weight loss diet plan.

The Intermittent Fasting Pyramid offers many advantages to help people lose weight effectively while boosting their health and wellbeing. But the diet program does limit calories several days each week, and it does require episodic food restriction, which may not be recommended in some instances. For example, individuals who have increased nutrient and calorie needs, and those who require a more regular dieting structure, would not be encouraged to implement intermittent fasting as a diet protocol. As always, it is important to first do no harm when considering a new diet program, and this is important when it comes to intermittent fasting as well.

## Individuals with High Calorie Needs

While the Intermittent Fasting Pyramid only encourages a modified fasting approach on its fasting day and transition days, it still limits caloric intake during this time. Therefore, as you can imagine, individuals with high calorie needs might be negatively affected during these fasting time periods. The following are known groups of individuals who fall into this category and should avoid intermittent fasting as a result.

- **Pregnant Women** – Women who are pregnant have extra caloric needs because they are not only meeting their own physical needs but those of their child as well. Restricting calories, even temporarily, is therefore not encouraged during pregnancy, and therefore, intermittent fasting is not a diet program appropriate for this group. Instead, consider other healthy diets rich in nutrients that can meet caloric needs in a more consistent and steady manner.

- **Women Who Are Breastfeeding** – Similar to pregnancy, breastfeeding requires both additional calories in the diet as well as consistent nutrition. Therefore, intermittent fasting should also be avoided if you are breastfeeding. Restricting calories and nutrients intermittently can affect the quality of breast milk and limit the child's access to full nutrition needed for healthy growth and development. Here again, choosing a healthy, well-balanced diet full of nutrition would be a better option.

- **Athletes with High Intensity Exercise Programs** – Exercising while using the Intermittent Fasting Pyramid is not something that needs to be avoided. In fact, regular physical activity and exercise are encouraged in your efforts to achieve a healthy weight and overall wellness. However, if you are an athlete or someone who has a high intensity exercise schedule, intermittent fasting might impact your performance during times where calories are being restricted. Appreciating this fact, other dieting plans might be preferable if you are concerned that fluctuations in your dieting might negatively affect your physical activity goals.

- **Children and Adolescents** – Throughout childhood and adolescence, growth and development are accelerated, and adequate nutrition is important. In addition to a well-balanced diet, an adequate and consistent number of calories are needed for kids and teens. Therefore, intermittent fasting is not considered a proper diet program for this group either. Once metabolism begins to slow in young adulthood, and calorie demands for growth and development are less, intermittent fasting may then be a good option for optimal health and weight control.

## Individuals with Concurrent Health Conditions

Individuals with select health conditions should also avoid intermittent fasting. The structure of the intermittent fasting regimen may trigger some specific health problems to worsen or become more difficult to manage. Therefore, intermittent fasting should also be avoided in these instances as well.

- **Individuals with Eating Disorders** – Anorexia, bulimia, binge-eating disorder, and other similar conditions represent a group of health conditions where intermittent fasting may pose challenges. Understanding that these disorders naturally involving periods where fasting, purging, or binging may exist, the structure of the Intermittent Fasting Pyramid could make these problems worse. In addition to seeking professional help and guidance, those who have these types of conditions, or who have had a history of an eating disorder, should avoid intermittent fasting regimens altogether.

- **People with Type I Diabetes** – In the previous chapter, intermittent fasting was offered as a consideration for individuals with Type II diabetes. Type II diabetics have actually been shown to develop better glucose control with reduced insulin resistance when using intermittent fasting diets.[38] However, all diabetic patients should discuss intermittent fasting with their physicians before starting, and those who have Type I diabetes should avoid intermittent fasting altogether. Specifically, for Type I diabetics, fasting periods may trigger hypoglycemic events while the return to a normal diet may cause them to "overshoot" their target glucose levels afterwards. Because of these risks, Type I diabetics should not try intermittent fasting as a dietary program. Individuals with type II diabetes should consult with their physician before trying intermittent fasting.

- **Individuals with High Stress/Anxiety** – While intermittent fasting offers weight loss and health advantages, it still imposes a mild stress on your body. If someone already has high levels of stress, or if they suffer from an anxiety, then adding intermittent fasting to the equation might not be ideal. In addition to having a higher risk of diet failure, your stress may worsen when reducing your caloric intake. Therefore, getting your anxiety under control first and/or effectively managing your stress is encouraged before you begin the Intermittent Fasting Pyramid.

## Additional Precautions with Intermittent Fasting

For the vast majority of people, intermittent fasting offers a great way to lose weight and boost your health. Likewise, the Intermittent Fasting Pyramid enhances these effects by making intermittent fasting less frustrating while reducing the risk of post-fast binge-eating. The conditions listed in this chapter identify some who should avoid intermittent fasting due to increased calorie and nutritional needs or due to concurrent illnesses that may respond poorly to fasting. If any doubt exists in this regard, consulting with a physician is strongly encouraged.

While the most common situations where intermittent fasting should be avoided have been listed, others may exist in individualized settings. For instance, people with chronic illnesses, immune disorders, or other health conditions may need to avoid fasting periods due to nutritional and calorie needs. If you have any health condition where this might be the case, getting professional advice from your health provider is similarly encouraged. But if none of these instances apply to you, intermittent fasting can actually be a means to prevent unwanted health conditions while maintaining a healthier weight.

SECTION V:

# The Program

# CHAPTER 11:

# Getting Started

So, you've decided to give the Intermittent Fasting Pyramid a try. Excellent! Regardless of whether you are choosing it for weight loss or for health reasons, or both, evidence clearly supports intermittent fasting as a great method for attaining wellness goals. And by using the Intermittent Fasting Pyramid, you increase your chances of success by making the diet easier to adopt with a better chance to keep the weight off. All you need to do now is a few things to make sure you get off on the right foot.

While the Intermittent Fasting Pyramid does not require a great deal of preparation, there are a few items that should be considered before starting your intermittent fasting schedule. For example, each of us have different caloric needs, which will affect the number of calories you are permitted during different days of the Intermittent Fasting Pyramid schedule. Likewise, you have choices regarding the type of dietary nutrition you'll want as well as the weekly schedule that is best for your lifestyle. Each of these will be discussed so that you can further improve your chances of success while using the Intermittent Fasting Pyramid.

## Step One – Determine Your Calorie Needs

Whenever you are trying to achieve a weight loss goal, knowing the number of calories your body requires each day just to maintain your current weight is important. As mentioned, this figure varies based on your gender, age, height, and level of activity, and therefore, determining your exact caloric needs is required in order for you to implement the Intermittent Fasting Pyramid effectively. Not only will this figure be required to determine the number of calories permitted during fasting and transitional days, but it will also be important to know during the regular meal days each week.

Understanding this, several daily calorie calculators can be used to determine your own personal needs. For example, the Mayo Clinic offers an easy-to-use calculator [https://www.mayoclinic.org/healthy-lifestyle/weight-loss/in-depth/calorie-calculator/itt-20402304] as do other reputable websites. Once you have identified your daily calorie needs, you will then use this figure to determine total caloric allowance during each day of the Intermittent Fasting Pyramid schedule. Knowing this figure will serve as your guide helping you stay on track and realize the wellness goals you want.

You can also manually calculate your daily calorie expenditure by multiplying your Basal Metabolic Rate (BMR) using the Harris-Benedict Equation and then multiplying that number by a factor based on your activity level. The equation is as follows:

*Men:*

*BMR = 66 + (6.2 × weight in pounds) + (12.7 × height in inches) – (6.76 age in years)*

*Women:*

$$BMR = 655.1 + (4.35 \times weight \; in \; pounds) + (4.7 \times height \; in \; inches) - (4.7 \times age \; in \; years)$$

Once you have your BRM from the above equation, multiply that number by the activity factor that best represents your activity level. That number will then provide you with your total calorie expenditure.

Multiply your BMR by one of the activity factors below.

Sedentary or light activity = 1.53

Active or moderately active = 1.76

Vigorously active = 2.25

## Step Two – Choose the Type of Nutritional Diet

One of the great things about intermittent fasting is that it can be used with a variety of diets if one prefers. For example, you may choose to simply eat a variety of foods without specific restrictions while just staying within the calorie limits set by the Intermittent Fasting Pyramid parameters.

Alternatively, however, you may select a specific diet to further enhance your health and wellbeing. While the latter is preferred from an overall health perspective, the flexibility of intermittent fasting does allow you to choose a diet that will best help you succeed in following your diet plan. For example, you may choose to obtain your daily caloric needs with a Mediterranean diet, a low-carb diet, a ketogenic diet or a vegan diet. As long as you stay within the guidelines of the Intermittent Fasting Pyramid from a calorie perspective, any of these and other traditional diets may be considered. Such a strategy may further enhance your overall wellness in the process.

## Step Three – Choose Your 7-Day Schedule

When describing the Intermittent Fasting Pyramid, it has been suggested that your fasting day be on Monday of each week. Subsequently, your transitional/partial fasting days would be on Tuesday and Wednesday. And of course, your regular meal days would be from Thursday through Sunday. The rationale for this approach is simply that many people will prefer to have a more regular eating pattern on the weekends simply from a social perspective. In other words, it would be easier to stick to your fasting regimen during the early part of the week when you might be less likely to be eating at restaurants or having scheduled social events.

While this type of Intermittent Fasting Pyramid schedule may be ideal for many people, it is certainly not an essential 7-day schedule that has to be adopted. Understanding this, you may benefit from arranging your fasting and transitional/partial fasting days on other days of the week depending on your own activities and schedule. It remains important that the two transitional/partial fasting days immediately follow your fasting day since this reduces the chances of post-fast binge-eating. But otherwise, feel free to arrange your Intermittent Fasting Pyramid however you like. And once a schedule is decided, simply stick to it so you can optimize your results.

The three steps listed are ones that are important to complete before you start your Intermittent Fasting Pyramid program. While the program has established calorie limits and a sequence of fasting, transitional and regular dieting, each of us have individual differences that will affect exactly how the Intermittent Fasting Pyramid should be implemented. By taking the time to complete these preparatory steps, you will increase your chances for success in reaching your weight loss and health goals.

In addition to these essential steps, you might want to consider a few other things before starting your Intermittent Fasting Pyramid. For one, all changes in dieting patterns benefit from various levels of support. This might be a friend or a family member, or it might be a local group that offers health support in general. This can be beneficial as well in helping you persevere as you adopt intermittent fasting as a healthy lifestyle approach.

Lastly, if you have any specific questions about whether intermittent fasting is right for you based on an existing health condition, be sure to check with your healthcare provider before starting the program. Several conditions may preclude starting the Intermittent Fasting Pyramid as previously discussed, but others may also exist. Therefore, it is better to be safe than sorry if you have any concerns about implementing intermittent fasting as a dietary program.

With these steps of preparation completed, you are now ready to begin your Intermittent Fasting Pyramid program. Soon, you will be on your way to better health and wellness while achieving a healthier weight and lifestyle.

*Ready, Set…Fast!*

# CHAPTER 12:

# Fasting Day

After preparing to begin your intermittent fasting program using the Intermittent Fasting Pyramid, your first day on your new diet will be your fasting day. Regardless whether you choose to start on a Monday or not, this will perhaps be the most challenging day of your week. But fortunately, with the Intermittent Fasting Pyramid, you don't have to completely avoid all food and calories. Instead, you are allowed roughly a quarter of your body's daily caloric needs. This will make this fasting day much more tolerable and much less frustrating.

When it comes to fasting, there are some general guidelines to help you achieve the dietary success you want. Likewise, additional measures can be used to make sure you feel as comfortable as possible while promoting positive health. In this chapter, we will briefly cover the parameters for your fasting day as part of the Intermittent Fasting Pyramid as well as some best practices to support your success. These suggestions will make sure you get off on the right foot and can better realize your weight loss and wellness goals.

## Fasting Day-The Basic Rules

As noted in the previous chapter on "Getting Started," determining your body's daily caloric needs is a necessary step so that you can calculate how many calories you are allowed during your fasting day. For example, if you determined your daily caloric needs are 2,000 calories a day, then you would permit yourself to eat 25 percent of this amount, or 500 calories, on your fasting day. If your daily caloric need is 2,200 calories a day, then you would consume 550 calories on your fasting day. By staying within this parameter, you will be able to reap the benefits of an intermittent fasting diet.

For most people, their fasting day calorie allowance will fall between 500 and 800 calories, although a few individuals may be allowed slightly less or slightly more. I do however suggest not going below 500 calories on your fasting day or 1,000 calories on your partial fasting days. If the 25% calculation puts you below the 500-calorie mark, simply stick to 500 calories. The same goes for the 50% calculation for your partial fasting days. If the calculation puts you below 1,000 calories, simply round up to 1,000 calories. In addition, you should also strive to go for a total of 14 to 16 hours without any caloric intake at all. For example, after the prior evening's dinner, you could avoid eating until the following day's lunch, which would allow 14 to 16 hours for complete fasting.

This fasting structure represents the ideal method for your fasting day while on the Intermittent Fasting Pyramid program. It limits your total number of calories for the entire fasting day to a quarter of your body's caloric needs. And it provides an extended period of time (approximately 14-16 hours) for complete fasting. Both of these measures have been shown to provide weight loss and health benefits, and therefore, this approach is encouraged as part of the Intermittent Fasting Pyramid.

## Additional Fasting Day Best Practices

As you can see, the overall structure for your fasting day is quite straightforward. But in addition to these simple parameters, there are some additional measures you can take to help make your fasting day more effective and comfortable. One of the most important best practices while fasting is making sure you stay well hydrated. Previously, we discussed how your body shifts over to ketosis during periods of fasting instead of glucose metabolism. Ketosis requires additional hydration since the level of ketone bodies in your body's circulation will rise during this time. Thus, it is quite important to drink plenty of water during your fasting day.

While water is important, other fluids may also serve as a means for hydration while also deterring your hunger. For example, black coffee and tea may be consumed during your fasting day. Both of these beverages provide some degree of hunger suppression while offering something pleasing to the palate. Also, sparkling water might be considered, which can be more pleasing and appealing than regular water during a fasting day. Finally, you may choose to engage in some activities that further help take your mind off your fast. Specifically, walking or meditating during your fasting day offers a method of distraction. Each of these activities and choices can be useful in helping you stay on track.

## Foods Selected During Your Fasting Day

As a final consideration, it is important to make good choices regarding the foods you eat during your fasting day. Even if your goal is to simply lose weight, choosing wholesome, nutritious foods will offer notable benefits. Why? Because choosing the right foods will make you feel better and provide you with more energy—making you more likely to stick to the plan. That is not to say you won't have some degree of hunger during your fasting day. But by choosing wholesome, nutritious foods for your restricted caloric meals, you will at least be giving your body essential vitamins, minerals, and nutrients that will help you feel your best.

By following these guidelines, and by implementing these recommended best practices, you will more easily tolerate your fasting day without difficulty. Given that you only need to complete one fasting day each week in the Intermittent Fasting Pyramid program, these strategies will make it easier for you to follow your plan and realize your wellness goals. And once your fasting day is done, the rest of the week will look so much more attractive!

# CHAPTER 13:

# Partial Fasting Days

Having completed your fasting day on the Intermittent Fasting Pyramid program, you next move onto your transitional or partial fasting days. These represent the next 2 days of your intermittent fasting plan, which have been suggested as being Tuesday and Wednesday after a Monday fast. Of course, you may choose a different weekly schedule that best fits your needs. Regardless, your two partial fasting days after your fasting day are quite important to your overall success.

The reason that partial fasting days are important is due to the fact that many people tend to over-eat or binge on the day or days following a fast. Having successfully accomplished their fasting day's calorie reduction, people often feel that they deserve a reward. Or they may simply over-eat in response to being hungry after their fast. In either case, post-fasting binges represent a major reason why many people struggle with intermittent fasting programs. But with the Intermittent Fasting Pyramid, these risks are significantly less likely to occur.

While partial fasting days in the Intermittent Fasting Pyramid account for its enhanced success rates, it remains important to follow specific parameters during these times. In this chapter, basic guidelines are provided for you to follow during your partial fasting days as well as typical best practices. These measures will again help ensure you stay on track as you move through the week and better achieve your weight loss and fitness goals.

## Partial Fasting Days – The Basic Rules

As part of the instructions provided for your fasting day in the Intermittent Fasting Pyramid program, it was recommended that you consume a quarter of your body's daily calorie needs. For your transitional or partial fasting days, this figure will be increased to half your body's daily calorie needs. As an example, for a person normally requiring 2,000 calories daily, they would consume only 1,000 calories during each of the partial fasting days. This figure would apply to Day 2 and Day 3 of your Intermittent Fasting Pyramid program. For the majority of people, the total number of calories allowed during partial fasting days on the Intermittent Fasting Pyramid will be between 1,000 to 1,200 calories.

Just remember, should your daily calorie needs calculation fall below 500 calories on your fasting day or below 1,000 on your partial fasting day, it is recommended that you adhere to no less than 500 calories on your fasting day and 1,000 calories on your partial fasting days. There is no reason to go below these two thresholds. For example if your daily calorie needs calculation came out to 1,500 calories a day, 25% of that number would be 375 calories. That number is too low and should be rounded up to a minimum of 500 calories.

Some individuals may have slightly less or slightly more caloric needs based on their age, gender, height, and activity levels. Therefore, you may require a slightly higher or lower number of calories during your partial fasting days. It should also be noted that having an extended period of time during each of the partial fasting days where no calories are consumed is preferred as part of the Intermittent Fasting Pyramid approach. By not eating after dinner the night before until lunchtime of each of the partial fasting days, you can achieve a complete fasting time of 14 to 16 hours. This strategy will boost weight loss as well as health outcomes if incorporated into your intermittent fasting plan.

As you likely appreciate, your partial fasting days are not nearly as intensive as your fasting day on the Intermittent Fasting Pyramid plan. And partial fasting days help deter any tendency to over-eat immediately after fasting by providing a clear structure for transitioning back to your normal diet. By gradually easing back into a regular dietary pattern, you will be more successful in attaining the weight loss you want. Simply abide by the partial fasting day structure during these two days, and your chances of success will be much greater.

## Additional Best Practices for Partial Fasting Days

In considering best practices for partial fasting days, many of the same recommendations outlined for your fasting day apply. Specifically, staying hydrated is important, and beverages like black coffee and tea can be used to help reduce your hunger. Similarly, taking walks and meditating can help you focus less on your hunger and more on other things. Lastly, choosing wholesome and nutritious foods for your partial fasting meals will provide your body with what it needs and improve both your mood and energy level. Each of these best practices will help you better adhere to your partial fasting days, which in turn will increase your ability to lose weight and become healthier over time.

Your partial fasting days represent the key to your ultimate success in using intermittent fasting to achieve weight loss and improve health. They are an essential part of the Intermittent Fasting Pyramid as these days will reduce the level of difficulty of an intermittent fasting diet while also making post-fast binge-eating less likely. These are key barriers that have prevented many from sticking with this healthy dietary lifestyle. But by employing these parameters and best practices during your partial fasting days, you will be more likely to overcome these challenges.

Notably, your approach to your partial fasting days is just as important as your approach to your fasting day itself. By taking partial fasting day strategies seriously, you give yourself a much better chance of weight loss and dietary success. This is where the Intermittent Fasting Pyramid clearly provides you with an advantage when compared to other intermittent fasting programs.

# CHAPTER 14:

# Non-Fasting Days

After completing your fasting day and your partial fasting days for the week, it's now time to return to your regular diet. For the next 4 days, you're not required to skip meals or go without food for any period of time. Doesn't that sound great?! Likewise, you can now eat the number of calories that your body and level of activity requires. This is the time you get to enjoy "life as usual." Therefore, by structuring your Intermittent Fasting Pyramid schedule correctly, these days will hopefully be times where you are more likely to socialize and dine outside your home.

While your non-fasting days have essentially no rules in terms of fasting requirements, there are still some best practices you should follow. After all, your ultimate goal is to lose weight and achieve better health. Therefore, the diet you choose as well as the lifestyle you lead during your non-fasting days can have a positive or negative impact on your overall success. As a result, we will explore some approaches that you might want to consider during your non-fasting days to improve your chances of adopting intermittent fasting as a long-term practice.

## Best Practices for Non-Fasting Days

During your non-fasting days, it is important to remember why you are intermittently fasting. Whether for weight loss or for better overall health, you decided to try the Intermittent Fasting Pyramid program for a reason. In addition to staying focused on these overall goals, the following are some additional best practices that are encouraged to foster greater success when adopting the Intermittent Fasting Pyramid plan.

- **Avoid Over-Compensating** – After completing your fasting day and partial fasting days, it is not uncommon to feel the urge to eat more than your body needs. In fact, this tendency probably has its roots in our ancient ancestors' experiences when they didn't know where or when their next meal would come. But in order to realize the benefits of the Intermittent Fasting Pyramid program fully, you should make sure your daily calories match what your body actually needs. In doing so, you will avoid undermining the gains you just made during the fasting portion of your program.

- **Choose Nutritious and Healthy Foods** – While your non-fasting days allow you to select any diet you like, foods that offer healthy nutrition and are wholesome in nature will provide you with more success. Certainly, intermittent fasting offers weight loss and health advantages regardless. But you can further improve these beneficial effects by eating healthy during non-fasting days as well. A number of healthy diet plans exist, and depending on your situation, several different ones might be considered. By trying to make good choices about the foods you eat all the time, you will be able to get the most out of your Intermittent Fasting Pyramid program.

- **Reward Yourself in Moderation** – Little rewards are important as motivations to stick to any diet. After all, you have committed to losing weight and becoming healthier, so a little "pat on the back" is well deserved. But rewarding yourself excessively can result in over-eating or undermining your overall health goals. Having a glass of wine or cocktail is certainly fine during your non-fasting days. And an occasional sweet or dessert offers a just reward for your efforts. But practice moderation in the process, and you will be much happier in the long run.

- **Stay Physically Active** – If you are looking to achieve weight loss or better health, staying active is another best practice to consider during your non-fasting days. In addition to being an appetite suppressant, exercise boosts your mental attitude and keeps you energized. This can help you stay on track with your Intermittent Fasting Pyramid plan and better prepare you for the week to follow.

- **Keep a Positive Outlook** – By adopting intermittent fasting as a dietary strategy to lose weight and be healthier, its focus is certainly on calorie intake and physical health. But at the same time, mental, emotional, and spiritual wellness is similarly important, and being healthy in these areas can increase your ability to get the most out of the Intermittent Fasting Pyramid approach. With this in mind, strive to keep a positive outlook while choosing activities and behaviors that offer holistic health. Doing so will offer many additional advantages you might not have expected.

## Gearing Up and Gearing Down

As a final thought regarding your non-fasting days during your Intermittent Fasting Pyramid program, the way you transition between the fasting portions and non-fasting portions of your dieting plan is important. For example, after your partial fasting days are completed, choose a smaller meal or snack as you begin your non-fasting days. And your final meals on your last non-fasting day each week should reduce portion size as the day proceeds. By "gearing up or down" at the beginning and end of your non-fasting period respectively, you will better tolerate these dietary transitions.

Overall, the behaviors and practices you choose to follow during your non-fasting days are up to you. None of the best practices are essential except avoiding any tendency to exceed your actual calorie needs on non-fasting days—something that should be easier due to the transitional or partial-fasting phase. But each of the recommendations listed can further improve your ability to maintain an intermittent fasting diet as a lifestyle while optimizing your results. This is where the advantages lie if you choose to incorporate them into your dieting strategy.

# CHAPTER 15:

# Intermittent Fasting Pyramid Meal Plan

One of the most difficult things to do when you start any new program is to determine what to eat. Although you can choose to develop your own meal plans, I wanted to provide you with a detailed plan to help get you started. Think of this three-week meal plan as your introduction to the Intermittent Fasting Pyramid. As you become more accustomed to the Intermittent Fasting Pyramid rules, it will be easy for you to develop your own meals and meal plans.

Just remember, everyone's caloric needs are unique so if you choose to follow the meal plans below, it's up to you to make sure you are sticking to the appropriate level of calories during your fasting and partial-fasting days. You may, therefore, need to increase or reduce your serving size depending on your specific calorie needs and your activity level.

I hope this detailed plan will help you get started. The recipes for the meals provided in the detailed meal plan can be found in Appendix I.

## Week 1 Meal Plan

### Day 1 (Fasting)
Breakfast: Skip breakfast (black coffee, water, tea or sparkling water until noon)
Lunch: Spinach, Pear and Walnut Salad
Dinner: Chicken and vegetable soup
*Note: No snacks on fasting days*

### Day 2 (Partial Fasting)
Breakfast: Skip breakfast (black coffee, water, tea or sparkling water until noon)
Lunch: Four Bean Salad
Snack: Apple and Almond Butter
Dinner: White Chicken Stew
*Note: A small snack is permissible on partial fasting days as long as you stay within your 50% calorie range.*

### Day 3 (Partial Fasting)
Breakfast: Skip breakfast (black coffee, water, tea or sparkling water until noon)
Lunch: White Chicken Stew (Left over from night before)
Snack: White Bean Hummus and Veggies
Dinner: Grilled Herb Chicken with Steamed Broccoli
*Note: A small snack is permissible on partial fasting days as long as you stay within your 50% calorie range.*

### Day 4 – 7 (Non-Fasting)
*No set meal-plan to follow but adhere to the non-fasting day rules.*
*Example of a non-fasting day*
Breakfast: Baked Egg and Avocado

Lunch: Greek Salad with Grilled Chicken
Snack: White Bean Hummus with Veggies and a glass of wine (optional)
Dinner: Vegetarian Chili

## Week 2 Meal Plan

### Day 1 (Fasting)
Breakfast: Skip breakfast (black coffee, water, tea or sparkling water until noon)
Lunch: Garden Salad with Grilled Chicken
Dinner: Grilled Halibut with Tomato, Avocado and Mango Salsa
*Note: No snacks on fasting days*

### Day 2 (Partial Fasting)
Breakfast: Skip breakfast (black coffee, water, tea or sparkling water until noon)
Lunch: Kale and Quinoa Salad
Snack: Greek Yogurt and Berries
Dinner: Shrimp Stir-Fry
*Note: A small snack is permissible on partial fasting days as long as you stay within your 50% calorie range.*

### Day 3 (Partial Fasting)
Breakfast: Skip breakfast (black coffee, water, tea or sparkling water until noon)
Lunch: Quinoa and Chickpea Salad
Snack: Celery with Almond Butter
Dinner: Ginger Salmon with Steamed Broccoli

*Note: A small snack is permissible on partial fasting days as long as you stay within your 50% calorie range.*

### Day 4 – 7 (Non-Fasting)
*No set meal plan to follow but adhere to the non-fasting day rules.*
*Example of a non-fasting day*
Breakfast: Berry Protein Smoothie
Lunch: Roasted Cauliflower and Spinach Salad
Snack: Trail Mix
Dinner: Almond Crusted Chicken with Roasted Vegetables and a glass of wine (optional)

## Week 3 Meal Plan

### Day 1 (Fasting)
Breakfast: Skip breakfast (black coffee, water, tea or sparkling water until noon)
Lunch: Garden Salad with Grilled Chicken
Dinner: Snapper en Papillote
*Note: No snacks on fasting days*

### Day 2 (Partial Fasting)
Breakfast: Skip breakfast (black coffee, water, tea or sparkling water until noon)
Lunch: White Bean and Asparagus Salad
Snack: Apple
Dinner: Quinoa Stuffed Peppers
*Note: A small snack is permissible on partial fasting days as long as you stay within your 50% calorie range*

## Day 3 (Partial Fasting)

Breakfast: Skip breakfast (black coffee, water, tea or sparkling water until noon)

Lunch: Quinoa Stuffed Peppers (Left over from night before)

Snack: 4 Strawberries

Dinner: Grilled Herb Chicken with Roasted Vegetables

*Note: A small snack is permissible on partial fasting days as long as you stay within your 50% calorie range*

## Day 4 – 7 (Non-Fasting)

*No set meal plan to follow but adhere to the non-fasting day rules.*

*Example of a non-fasting day*

Breakfast: Strawberry Coconut Chia Bowl

Lunch: Spaghetti Squash with Fresh Herbs

Snack: Apple and Almond Butter

Dinner: Salmon and Pepper Stir-Fry and a glass of wine (optional)

# SECTION VI:

# You Can Do It!

# CHAPTER 16:

# **Staying Motivated**

When it comes to dieting, it is often quoted that 9 out of every 10 people who try to diet end up gaining the weight back, or worse, weighing even more than they did originally. While these statistics are somewhat exaggerated, it is fair to say that more than half who start a diet end up "falling off the wagon." In some cases, the diet they selected becomes bland and unpalatable. In other instances, a lack of time to properly plan meals undermines their diet's success. But by far, most diets fail simply because of challenges sustaining motivation.

Fortunately, strategies to maintain a higher level of motivation can be used to improve your chances of success. These strategies can help you in your motivation for any diet, but they are specifically beneficial when it comes to intermittent fasting. For the 40 percent of the world's population who will diet at some point in their lives, this is great news. By employing a few simple techniques, you will be much more likely to reach your weight loss and health objectives. And combining these techniques with the Intermittent Fasting Pyramid program increases this likelihood even more.

## Understanding Human Motivation

What exactly is it that keeps us motivated when pursuing a goal? In terms of dieting, most people's objectives can be assumed to be weight loss and better health, which certainly seem like desirable targets. Based on this alone, it would seem like this would be enough to stay motivated. But as noted, failures to stick to a diet are very common. Therefore, it is clear that a high level of sustained motivation requires more than just an important goal. The goal also has to be realistic and achievable, and we need to believe that we are personally capable of reaching the goal.

Whenever we identify something we want to achieve, each of us go through a process of analyzing the costs versus benefits. In other words, are the advantages of attaining the goal actually worth the time, energy, and effort it takes to get there? When it comes to weight loss and health goals, most of us assign significant value to these goals, and therefore, the benefit is usually assumed to be rather high. After all, millions of people wouldn't pursue weight loss each year if it wasn't something that most of us thought was valuable. So, assuming the advantages of weight loss are high for most of us, the costs of sticking to the diet are often key factors that cause us to lose motivation.

When we examine these costs, dieting can certainly demand a great deal of us. It requires time to plan meals and educate ourselves about a particular diet. Likewise, transitioning from our regular eating patterns to a new dietary plan is stressful. From hunger, to changes in energy levels, to changes in our grocery lists, notable barriers exist when it comes to "sticking to the plan." As we become increasingly aware of these difficulties, we begin to question whether our efforts are worth it. This can certainly be a stumbling block that causes many of us to give up on our efforts.

Motivation can be affected by another factor besides the costs we experience in dieting. Even if our struggle is relatively mild and the costs rather minimal, motivation can begin to fade if we fail to see the results we are expecting. Requiring "proof" that what we are doing is producing positive results is simply a part of human nature. If our weight is not changing, or not changing as quickly as we expect, we begin to question the diet or the way we are pursuing it. And understandably, this might be a good reason to reevaluate things. But when expectations are not realistic, or when a lack of knowledge about a diet's weight loss effects is inaccurate, then we lose faith before a diet might have a chance to work.

Motivation can therefore be affected by a variety of factors. Despite being highly motivated to lose weight and start a diet plan, our commitment can weaken in time when our efforts don't seem worth the effort or when a lack of positive feedback is being recognized. And these factors can often carry greater weight when they are poorly aligned to realistic expectations. However, there are several techniques that can be employed to help you keep a high level of motivation while dieting. And while this is helpful for any type of dieting, these approaches are certainly beneficial when combined with the Intermittent Fasting Pyramid program.

## Intermittent Fasting–Best Practices for Staying Motivated

When we start a new diet, we're usually excited, energized, and motivated to succeed. We cannot wait to embrace our new lifestyle and eating habits to be more fit and healthy. Wouldn't it be nice to maintain this level of excitement and passion all the way through? While some let-down in your enthusiasm is to be expected, that doesn't mean you have to lose your momentum. With the following best practices you can stay motivated and improve your chances of success.

- **Educate Yourself and Have Realistic Expectations** – Wouldn't it be great if there were a diet that allowed us to lose 20 pounds a week without any difficulty at all? Such a diet might alleviate some of the motivational challenges we often experience since it would provide both great feedback and help us quickly reach our weight loss goals. In reality, however, we have to align expectations with what is most likely to occur. For example, with intermittent fasting, weight loss is moderate in nature and extended over a longer period of time. Thus, it is important to appreciate that intermittent fasting using the Intermittent Fasting Pyramid is more of a lifestyle change than a temporary weight loss diet. By learning about intermittent fasting and the typical weight loss you can expect, you are less likely to be disillusioned and lose motivation when your expectations and reality fail to align.

- **Make Several "Small" Goals Leading to Your "Big" Goal** – Whenever you commit to a long-term goal, you can increase your level of persistence by "stair-stepping" your way there. In other words, establishing a series of smaller goals leading up your ultimate target helps you stay on track. Why? Simply because this allows you to see positive feedback and feel that your efforts are worthwhile and making a difference. Therefore, with intermittent fasting, you should create biweekly targets that are reasonable and that support your efforts. This will certainly help you stay motivated along the way.

- **Make a Plan that Fits Your Lifestyle** – Sometimes we lose motivation when our diet plan simply doesn't fit into our life's schedule. Sticking to a diet is hard enough, but when our lifestyle makes this even more difficult, the chance that our motivation dwindles is pretty high. That's the reason that the schedule you select for your fasting and partial fasting days is important. While the Intermittent Fasting Pyramid makes intermittent fasting less cumbersome, you can still do yourself a favor by aligning your 7-day schedule with what works best for your lifestyle. Doing so will remove one additional obstacle that could hinder your motivation over time.

- **Know (and Revisit Often) Your Motivations** – Why did you think about dieting in the first place? Was it to lose weight or lower your blood pressure? Perhaps you were motivated for an upcoming high school reunion or by an old picture of yourself from 10 years ago. No matter what your motivations for dieting might be, it is important to list them, recite them, and constantly remind yourself what they are. In fact, picture boards that help you visualize these motivations and personal goals should be created and placed where you will frequently see them. This helps you keep your incentives fresh in your mind (and sight), which can help you persevere when you're having a tough day.

- **Enlist Support for Success** – Having friends and family members support you in your health efforts is a good idea for two reasons. First, having others support our efforts helps us stick to the plan. If others know our intentions, they can help us by not offering us foods that undermine our diet. Secondly, having others aware of our plans for intermittent fasting (as well as our goals) holds us accountable to someone beside ourselves. Not only will we not want to let ourselves down, but we won't want to let them down either. For these reasons, social supports are strongly recommended to help keep a higher level of motivation when on the Intermittent Fasting Pyramid program.

- **Use Small Rewards to Push You Forward** – As part of your motivational plan, you now appreciate the importance of setting smaller goals along the way in reaching your ultimate goal of weight loss and better health. An additional strategy to keep your level of motivation high is to reward yourself each time you reach these smaller goals. This little "prize" can lift your spirits and give you a boost that might be just what you need at the time. These smaller rewards are a great way to help you stay focused and maintain a higher level of motivation. Just remember, rewards don't have to be food related. It can be a new bathing suit or pair of pants in a smaller size or even a small reward like a new water bottle.

## The Intermittent Fasting Pyramid as a Lifestyle Choice

The motivation strategies listed in this chapter can be used whenever you are pursuing a health goal. But they work quite well with the Intermittent Fasting Pyramid program. As you adopt your new 7-day intermittent fasting schedule, these techniques can help you stay motivated and focused week after week. And by adopting as many of these strategies as possible, you will naturally be more likely to lose the weight you want over time.

While you may choose to use the Intermittent Fasting Pyramid program for a limited time to reach your weight loss and health goals, you may also wish to adopt intermittent fasting as a long-lasting lifestyle change. As noted, intermittent fasting offers many health advantages when practiced regularly. This, and the fact the Intermittent Fasting Pyramid program is a diet that is better tolerated than most, makes it a reasonable long-term option.

If you choose to adopt the Intermittent Fasting Pyramid program as a lifestyle diet, you will still need to practice motivational strategies until intermittent fasting becomes a habit and normal way of eating. Though the precise amount of time required for this may vary slightly, it generally takes three weeks to acquire a new habit. Understanding this, the motivation strategies in this chapter should be used for at least this length of time to help you get well accustomed to an intermittent fasting lifestyle. By that time, it is very likely you will be on your way to realizing your weight loss and health goals and will want to persevere even without these motivational techniques.

# CHAPTER 17

# Customizing the Intermittent Fasting Pyramid

We are all extremely unique. And that uniqueness determines how quickly we lose weight, how motivated we are and even our expectations of a new diet or weight loss plan.

The intermittent Fasting Pyramid can be an intense program for many. And if you only have a few pounds to lose and are not experiencing any of the negative health consequences we discussed in the beginning of the book, you may not need to be as strict with your intermittent fasting.

Here are two modifications that allow you to customize the your Intermittent Fasting Pyramid.

## Modification #1

Who is this customization for? The first modification is for anyone who is losing weight too quickly or doesn't have a lot of weight to lose.

In this scenario, you can take out one of the partial fasting days. So your pyramid will now look like this:

> *Day One: Fasting Day (25% of your daily caloric needs)*

*Day Two: Partial Fasting Day (50% of your daily caloric needs)*
*Day Three – Seven: Non-Fasting Days*

## Modification #2

Who is this customization for?

This second modification is for anyone who finds the fasting day too intense. That is, they become dizzy, nauseous, lightheaded or generally unwell during their fasting day. Fasting days are typically difficult for all—especially when you are just starting out—but some people can have more intense side effects. If you are experiencing any of the above, this modification would be a better choice for you.

In this scenario, you take out your fasting day and simply go right to your partial fasting days. So your pyramid will now look like this:

*Day One and Two: Partial Fasting Days (50% of your daily caloric needs)*
*Day Three – Seven: Non-Fasting Days*

Don't be afraid to modify your Intermittent Fasting Pyramid so it works best for you. Even with this modification, you will still reap the benefits of weight loss and better health.

# CHAPTER 18:

# The 3-Week Online Challenge

Want a little extra motivation to help you get started and stick to the plan? Join me and take the 3-week Intermittent Fasting Pyramid Online Challenge. With the online challenge, you will have everything you need to succeed and I will personally be your guide on this incredible journey.

As part of the 3-week Intermittent Fasting Pyramid Online Challenge, you will receive the following:

Three video tutorials

- Welcome Video
- What is the Intermittent Fasting Pyramid?
- Getting Started

Detailed and easy-to-follow meal plans

- Week 1 Meal Plan
- Week 2 Meal Plan
- Week 3 Meal Plan

Shopping lists

- Week 1 Shopping List

- Week 2 Shopping List
- Week 3 Shopping List

Intermittent Fasting Pyramid Recipes (with photos)
Intermittent Fasting Pyramid: The Rules
The Beginner's Guide to the Intermittent Fasting Pyramid

Plus, two incredible bonuses!

- 27 Detox Water Recipes
- 10 Best Smoothies

Go to www.DawnaStone.com/IntermittentFasting

# Pyramid Fasting Recipes

## BONUS RECIPES

* These select recipes are from my *Healthy You Diet* cookbook. Although only a few of the recipes from my *Healthy You Diet* cookbook are included in the Intermittent Fasting Pyramid program many of the 100+ recipes in the cookbook would make great low calorie options for your fasting and partial fasting days. You can find the cookbook on Amazon or go to DawnaStone.com for a direct link to the Amazon page.

# Almond Crusted Chicken

## Ingredients:

¾ cup almond meal

¼ cup oat flour

¼ teaspoon paprika

¼ teaspoon cayenne pepper

½ teaspoon onion powder

½ teaspoon oregano

2 teaspoons sea salt

½ teaspoon garlic powder

2 eggs

4 boneless, skinless chicken breasts

2 tablespoons extra-virgin olive oil

## Directions:

In a large bowl, combine the almond meal, oat flour, paprika, onion powder, oregano, salt and garlic powder and set aside.

In a medium bowl, whisk the eggs and set aside.

Pound the chicken to an even thickness (about ½ inch) by placing the breasts between 2 plastic bags or sheets of plastic wrap and hitting the thick part of the chicken with a flat meat pounder or rolling pin.

Dip the chicken breasts into the egg mixture. After dipping

chicken into the egg, dip into the dry mixture so that it is evenly covered.

In a deep skillet, heat the oil on medium-high heat. Add the chicken to the skillet and cook for 6 to 8 minutes on each side or until cooked through. Time will depend on the thickness of the chicken.

Makes 4 servings

# Baked Egg and Avocado

## Ingredients:

1 ripe avocado, halved and pitted
2 eggs
½ teaspoon sea salt
¼ teaspoon black pepper

## Directions:

Preheat oven to 425°F.

To allow room for the egg, scoop out an additional tablespoon or two from the center of each avocado half.

Place avocado on a small baking dish lined with parchment paper and crack an egg into each half.

Bake for 15-20 minutes or until egg whites have set and yolk is still runny. Remove from oven and add salt and pepper.

Makes 2 servings

# Berry Protein Smoothie*

## Ingredients:

1 scoop high quality pea protein powder
1 cup unsweetened plain almond milk
½ cup frozen berries (strawberries, blackberries and/or blueberries)
2 ice cubes

## Directions:

In a blender, combine pea protein powder, almond milk, berries and ice.

Makes 1 serving

*This recipe is from my Healthy You Diet cookbook. You can find out more or get the link to Amazon at DawnaStone.com

# Chicken and Vegetable Soup

## Ingredients:

1 tablespoon extra virgin olive oil
½ onion diced
1 clove garlic
2 carrots, sliced
4 cups chicken broth
1 can diced tomatoes
4 celery stalks, sliced
1 zucchini, spiralized or chopped
2 cups spinach, stems removed
1 rotisserie chicken breast, shredded (already cooked)

## Directions:

Heat the oil in a Dutch oven medium-high heat. Add the onion
and garlic, stirring frequently for 3-4 minutes or until the onion
is translucent. Add the carrots and stir for 1 minute. Add the
broth, canned tomatoes, celery and zucchini. Bring to a boil,
reduce heat and simmer for 12-15 minutes or until vegetables
are tender. Add the spinach and shredded chicken and simmer
for an additional 10 minutes.

Makes 2 servings

# Four-Bean Salad

## Ingredients:

### Salad:
2 cups yellow wax beans, cut in half and trimmed
2 cups green beans, cut in half and trimmed
4 radishes, washed and sliced thin
1 cup garbanzo beans
1 cup northern beans (or any white bean)
¼ cup roughly chopped fresh dill

### Dressing:
½ cup extra virgin olive oil
¼ cup white balsamic vinegar
½ teaspoon sea salt
¼ teaspoon ground black pepper

## Directions:

For the dressing, whisk together the vinegar, oil, salt and pepper in a medium bowl and set aside (or use any of the dressings in this appendix).

In a large pot with a tight-fitting lid, place a steamer tray in the pot and add enough cold water to cover the bottom of the pot by about 1-2 inches. Cover the pot and bring the water to a boil. Add the yellow and green beans and lower the heat to a simmer. Steam the vegetables to a tender-crisp and take care not to overcook.

While the vegetables are steaming prepare an ice bath (large bowl of water with ice cubes). When the vegetables are done, drain with a strainer and immediately place in the ice bath. Once cooled, remove from ice bath and set aside.

In a large bowl combine yellow beans, green beans, radishes, garbanzo beans, northern beans, and dill. Gently mix, top with dressing and serve.

Makes 4 servings

# Garden Salad with Grilled Chicken

## Ingredients:

1 boneless, skinless chicken breast (organic or hormone-free preferred)
Pinch of salt
Pinch of ground black pepper
2 cups romaine lettuce, torn into bite-size pieces
1 small tomato, sliced
4 thin slices, red onion
¼ cucumber, sliced
1 tablespoons white balsamic vinaigrette (see recipe in dressing section)

## Directions:

Prepare grill, or preheat broiler. Season chicken with salt and pepper. Grill or broil chicken for 15-20 minutes, turning once or until no trace of pink remains. Cut chicken into strips.

Wash and place salad and remaining ingredients in bowl and toss with dressing. Top with chicken.

Makes 1 serving

# Ginger Salmon

## Ingredients:

1 teaspoon fresh ginger, minced
2 tablespoons reduced-sodium soy sauce or tamari (gluten-free/wheat-free)*
2 (4-oz) salmon fillets, skin removed
Extra virgin olive oil spray
1 teaspoon toasted sesame seeds

## Directions:

Combine ginger and soy sauce in large sealable plastic bag. Add fish, and shake gently to coat. Place in refrigerator. Preheat broiler. Place fish on broiler pan coated with cooking spray. Broil 13-15 minutes, or until fish flakes easily with fork.

Sprinkle with sesame seeds.

Makes 2 servings

# Greek Salad with Grilled Chicken

## Ingredients:

2 boneless, skinless chicken breasts
Salt, to taste
Pepper, to taste
4 cups romaine lettuce, torn into bite-size pieces
1 tomato, sliced
8-10 Kalamata olives
½ cucumber, seeded and chopped
¼ cup red onion, finely chopped
¼ cup feta cheese, crumbled (optional)
2 tablespoons Greek dressing (see recipe in dressing section)

## Directions:

Prepare grill or preheat broiler. Season chicken with salt and pepper. Grill or broil chicken for 15-20 minutes, turning once, or until no trace of pink remains. Cut chicken into strips.

Combine lettuce, tomato, olives, cucumber, and red onion in large bowl. Sprinkle with feta and toss with Greek dressing. Top with chicken and serve.

Makes 2 servings

# Greek Vinaigrette (Dressing)

## Ingredients:

¼ cup extra virgin olive oil

2 tablespoons red wine vinegar

2 tablespoons fresh oregano, chopped or 1 tablespoon dried

1 tablespoon feta, crumbled (optional*)

½ teaspoon sea salt

¼ teaspoon black pepper

## Directions:

In a small jar (with lid) or bowl mix together the oil and vinegar.
Add oregano, feta, salt and pepper and mix well.

Makes approximately ½ cup

# Greek Yogurt with Fresh Berries

## Ingredients:

1 cup Greek yogurt (or non-dairy yogurt)
3 strawberries, sliced

## Directions:

In a bowl, top Greek yogurt with berries and enjoy!

Makes 1 serving

# Grilled Halibut with Tomato, Avocado and Mango Salsa*

## Ingredients:

**Salsa**

½ tomato, seeded and diced
½ cup ripe mango, peeled and diced (optional*)
¼ cups red onion, finely chopped
¼ cup fresh cilantro, chopped
2 tablespoons freshly squeezed lime juice
¼ teaspoon salt
Ground black pepper to taste

**Fish**

2 (4 oz) halibut filets
½ tablespoon extra virgin olive oil
Salt
Pepper
1 lime

## Directions:

In medium bowl, combine first 7 tomato-mango salsa ingredients, and let stand for 15 to 20 minutes.

Preheat grill or broiler, lightly brush halibut with olive oil, and season with salt and pepper. Place fish on grill or in broiler. Cook 5 to 7 minutes per side (make sure fish is opaque at its center).

Top fish with salsa and serve.

Makes 2 servings

*This recipe is from my Healthy You Diet cookbook. You can find out more or get the link to Amazon at* DawnaStone.com

# Grilled Herb Chicken*

## Ingredients:

4 boneless, skinless chicken breasts (organic or hormone-free preferred)
1 tablespoon extra virgin olive oil
1 teaspoon dried oregano
1 teaspoon thyme
1 teaspoon rosemary
½ teaspoon salt
¼ teaspoon garlic, minced

## Directions:

Preheat grill on medium heat. Lightly oil grates so chicken doesn't stick. Rinse chicken, and place in large re-sealable plastic bag with olive oil. Seal, and shake. Open bag, and add ingredients. Shake bag to coat chicken. Cook chicken approximately 7-10 minutes on each side, or until thoroughly cooked.

Note: If you don't have access to a grill, place chicken in a grill pan.

Makes 4 servings

*This recipe is from my Healthy You Diet cookbook. You can find out more or get the link to Amazon at DawnaStone.com

# Kale and Quinoa Salad*

## Ingredients:

**Salad:**
¾ cup red quinoa
1 ½ cup water
1 teaspoon salt
½ bunch kale, washed, stems removed and chopped
1 carrot, chopped
1 tomato, chopped
½ cucumber, chopped
½ yellow pepper, chopped
¼ red onion, chopped
1 tablespoon sliced almonds

**Dressing** (or use any of the dressing recipes in this appendix)
½ cup extra virgin olive oil
1 tablespoon balsamic vinegar
1 teaspoon salt
¼ teaspoon black pepper
1 teaspoon Dijon mustard

## Directions:

Combine quinoa, water and salt in a saucepan. Bring to a boil, reduce heat and simmer on low until water is absorbed (approximately 15 minutes). Remove from heat and keep covered.

To make the dressing, whisk together olive oil, balsamic vinegar, salt, pepper and Dijon mustard in a small bowl and set aside.

In a large bowl combine kale, carrots, tomato, cucumber, pepper and onion. Fold in the quinoa and gently stir.

Split between two bowls, sprinkle with sliced almonds and drizzle with dressing.

Make 2 servings

*\*This recipe is from my Healthy You Diet cookbook. You can find out more or get the link to Amazon at* DawnaStone.com

# Quinoa and Chickpea Salad

## Ingredients:

### Salad:

½ cup quinoa
½ cup chickpeas
½ cup red kidney beans
1 carrot, sliced thin
2 celery stalks, sliced thin
1 teaspoon sea salt

### Dressing:

2 tablespoon extra virgin olive oil
1 tablespoon balsamic vinegar
½ teaspoon sea salt
¼ teaspoon black pepper
½ teaspoon dried oregano

## Directions:

Cook quinoa according to package directions. Cover and refrigerate until chilled.

Add the chickpeas, beans, carrots, celery, and sea salt to the quinoa and toss to mix.

In a small bowl, whisk together the olive oil, balsamic vinegar, sea salt, black pepper, and oregano. Pour the dressing over the quinoa mixture and toss well to combine. The salad can be stored in the refrigerator for 2 to 3 days. You can also choose any of the salad dressing recipes in this appendix.

Makes 2 servings

# Quinoa Stuffed Peppers

## Ingredients:

1 ½ cups quinoa
3 cups vegetable broth
1 tablespoon extra virgin olive oil, plus more for preparing baking pan
½ small yellow onion, diced
1 large carrot, diced
2 cloves garlic, minced
1 teaspoon cumin
1 teaspoon dried oregano
1 teaspoon sea salt
½ teaspoon black pepper
1/3 cup sliced almonds
4 red or yellow bell peppers, cored, seeded and halved (reserve top of pepper)

## Directions:

Preheat the oven to 400°F.

In a saucepan over medium-high heat, combine the quinoa and broth and bring to a boil. Reduce the heat to low, cover, and cook for about 15 minutes, or until the broth is absorbed. Fluff with a fork and set aside.

In a Dutch oven over medium-high heat, heat the oil. Add the onion and cook, stirring frequently, for 4 to 5 minutes, or until translucent. Add the carrots, and garlic, and cook stirring frequently for 1 minute. Add the reserved quinoa, cumin, oregano, salt, pepper, and almonds and cook for 1 to 2 minutes more. Set aside to let filling cool until slightly warm.

Oil a 9×12 baking pan. Divide the quinoa mixture evenly among the bell peppers. Place the reserved top on each pepper and arrange them upright in the pan. Cover the peppers with foil and bake for approximately 30-40 minutes or until peppers are tender and filling is hot throughout. Transfer to plates and serve.

Makes 4 servings

# Roasted Cauliflower and Spinach Salad

## Ingredients:

1 head cauliflower, cut into bite-size pieces
2 tablespoons extra virgin olive oil
2 teaspoon sea salt
2 cups spinach, stems removed
1 carrot, chopped
2 dates, pitted and chopped
1 tablespoon pine nuts

### Dressing:
¼ cup olive oil
1 tablespoon balsamic vinegar
½ teaspoon sea salt
¼ teaspoon

## Directions:

Preheat oven to 400 degrees. Place cauliflower on a baking tray and drizzle with extra virgin olive oil. Add salt.

Roast for 12-15 minutes or until cauliflower is tender.

In a small bowl, whisk together olive oil, vinegar, salt and pepper and set aside.

In a medium to large bowl, combine spinach, carrots, dates and pine nuts. Top with roasted cauliflower and toss with dressing

Makes 2 servings

# Roasted Vegetables (side)

## Ingredients:

6-10 small carrots, yellow, purple and orange, sliced lengthwise
½ pound Brussels spouts, sliced in half
½ red onion, sliced
1-2 tablespoon extra virgin olive oil
1 teaspoon sea salt
½ teaspoon ground black pepper

## Directions:

Pre-heat oven to 400 degrees. Place all ingredients on a baking tray and drizzle with extra virgin olive oil. Add salt and pepper.

Bake for 15-20 minutes or until vegetables are tender.

Makes 2 servings

# Salmon and Bell Pepper Stir Fry

## Ingredients:

### Sauce
1 teaspoon honey (optional)
2 tablespoons tamari
2 tablespoons vegetable stock

### Stir-Fry
2 tablespoons sesame oil
1 pound salmon fillet
1 clove garlic, minced
3 bell peppers (yellow, orange and red), seeded and sliced
2 teaspoon minced ginger
1 teaspoon sesame seeds

## Directions:

*To make the sauce:* In a small bowl, combine honey, tamari, and vegetable stock and mix well. Set aside.

*To make the stir-fry:* In a large skillet over medium-high heat, heat the oil and swirl the pan to coat. Cook salmon for 2 minutes on each side (salmon will not be completely done). Remove salmon and set aside. Add garlic to the pan stirring consistently for 1 to 2 minutes. Add bell peppers and pour on reserved sauce mixture and cook, stirring constantly, for 3 to 4 minutes. Add ginger and reserved salmon and cook for an additional 2 to 3 minutes or until salmon is done and bell peppers are tender. Sprinkle with sesame seeds and serve.

Makes 4 servings

# Shrimp Stir-Fry

## Ingredients:

### Sauce
2 tablespoons tamari
2 tablespoons vegetable stock

### Stir-Fry
¾ cup quinoa, rinsed and drained (optional)
1.5 cups water (optional)
2 tablespoons sesame oil
1 pound medium shrimp, peeled and deveined
2 green onions, chopped
1 clove garlic, minced
½ head cabbage, chopped or shredded
2/3 cup shredded carrots
2 cups snow peas
2 teaspoon minced ginger

## Directions:

*To make the sauce:* In a small bowl, combine the tamari, and vegetable stock and mix well. Set aside.

*To make the quinoa (optional):* In a saucepan over medium-high heat, combine the quinoa and water and bring to a boil. Reduce the heat to low, cover, and cook for 15 minutes, or until the water is absorbed. Set aside, covered, to steam for 5 minutes. Fluff the quinoa with a fork and transfer to a bowl. Set aside.

*To make the stir-fry:* In a large skillet over medium-high heat, heat the oil and swirl the pan to coat. Cook shrimp for 1 minute on each side (shrimp will not be completely done). Remove shrimp and set aside. Add onions and garlic to the pan stirring consistently for 1 to 2 minutes. Add cabbage, carrots, and snow peas, and pour on reserved sauce mixture and cook, stirring constantly, for 2 to 3 minutes. Add ginger and shrimp and cook for an additional 2 to 3 minutes or until shrimp is done.

Fluff the reserved quinoa with a fork and divide it among 4 plates. Spoon the stir-fry mixture over the quinoa and serve.

Makes 4 servings

*Eliminate quinoa if eating on a fasting or transition day.

# Snapper and Asparagus en Papillote*

## Ingredients:

2 1/2 cups water
4 (4 oz) snapper or halibut fillets
Sea salt
Ground black pepper
1 tablespoon extra-virgin olive oil
24 thin asparagus spears, trimmed
1 lemon, thinly sliced
2 tablespoons chopped fresh dill or flat-leaf parsley, or 1 1/2 teaspoons dried dill

## Directions:

Preheat the oven to 375°F.

Cut 4 sheets of parchment paper, each approximately 18" × 12".

Fold the parchment in half the long way. Using scissors, cut a large heart out of each piece of paper, beginning the cut on the fold.

Season both sides of the fish lightly with salt and pepper. Place 1 fillet on one half of a parchment heart, leaving at least a 1" border. Drizzle with one-quarter of the oil and top with 6 asparagus spears and a few lemon slices. Sprinkle with one-quarter of the dill or parsley. Fold the other side of the heart over the fish and twist the edges together to make a seal. Fold the bottom edge under the packet to keep it from opening during cooking. Repeat with the remaining ingredients.

Transfer the packets to 2 baking sheets and bake for 12 to 15 minutes. Using oven mitts or tongs, transfer the packets to 4 plates. Be sure everyone is at the table to open their packet with scissors. Take care because the steam is hot. Serve with the rice.

Makes 4 servings

*\*This recipe is from my Healthy You Diet cookbook. You can find out more or get the link to Amazon at* DawnaStone.com

# Spaghetti Squash with Fresh Herbs

## Ingredients:

1 medium spaghetti squash
1 tablespoon extra virgin olive oil
1 clove garlic, minced
1 medium tomato, chopped
1 tablespoon fresh basil, minced
¼ cup pine nuts
¼ cup grated Parmesan cheese (optional*)
sea salt
pepper

## Directions:

Pre-heat the oven to 375°F.

Pierce the squash in several places with a fork. Microwave whole squash on high for 10 minutes. Place whole squash on glass baking sheet and roast for 1 hour or until tender.

Let cool for 5 to 10 minutes, cut in half lengthwise and scrape the insides with a fork to remove the long strands of flesh. Transfer to a bowl.

In a skillet, heat 1 tablespoon olive oil over medium heat. Add garlic and sauté for 1 minute. Add tomatoes and sauté for 1 minute. Turn off heat and add spaghetti squash, basil, oregano and salt. Gently combine ingredients.

Divide between two bowls and top with pine nuts and cheese and salt and pepper to taste.

Makes 2 servings

# Spinach, Pear and Walnut Salad*

## Ingredients:

4 cups baby spinach
1/2 fennel bulb, thinly sliced
1 pear, cored, peeled, and thinly sliced
1/4 cup coarsely chopped walnuts
1/4 cup thinly sliced red onion
1/4 cup sliced button mushrooms
2 tablespoons raisins
1/4 cup Walnut Vinaigrette (page 163)

## Directions:

In a salad bowl, combine the spinach, fennel, pear, walnuts, onion, mushrooms, and raisins.

Add the vinaigrette and toss just before serving.

Makes 2 servings

*This recipe is from my Healthy You Diet cookbook. You can find out more or get the link to Amazon at DawnaStone.com

# Strawberry Coconut Chia Bowl

## Ingredients:

### Pudding:
1 tablespoon chia seeds
1 cup almond milk
1 cup plain full fat Greek yogurt (or nondairy option)
1 tablespoon honey (or maple syrup)

### Topping:
4 strawberries, sliced
1 tablespoon sliced almonds
1 tablespoon unsweetened coconut flakes
1 teaspoon flax seeds

## Directions:

Mix pudding ingredients and refrigerate for at least 30-45 minutes (or overnight). Top with strawberries, almonds, coconut and flax and enjoy!

Makes 1 serving

# Steamed Asparagus (side)

## Ingredients:

1 bunch asparagus

## Directions:

Clean and cut asparagus. Bring 1 inch water and salt to boil in saucepan with steamer. Add asparagus, and cover, reduce heat to medium, and cook for 4-6 minutes, or until asparagus is bright green and tender.

Makes 2 servings

# Steamed Broccoli (side)

## Ingredients:

1 head broccoli

## Directions:

Rinse broccoli, cut off stalk, and break into bite-size pieces. Bring 1-inch water and salt to boil in saucepan with steamer. Add broccoli, and cover, reduce heat to medium, and cook for 4-6 minutes, or until broccoli is bright green and tender.

Makes 4 servings

# Trail Mix (snack)

## Ingredients:

1 tablespoon dried cherries
1 tablespoon raw pumpkin seeds
1 tablespoon sliced almonds
4 dried apricots, sliced
1 tablespoon coconut
2 figs, quartered

## Directions:

In a small bowl, combine cherries, pumpkin seeds, almonds, apricots, coconut, and figs. Place in a jar or sealable bag and have ready for snacking.

Makes 2 servings

# Vegetarian Chili

## Ingredients

1 tablespoon extra-virgin olive oil
½ red onion, finely chopped
1 clove garlic, minced
2 stalks celery, chopped
1 teaspoon chili powder
1 teaspoon cumin
1 teaspoon ground coriander
½ teaspoon sea salt
1 cup crushed tomatoes
1 cup water
1 cup garbanzo beans, cooked and drained
1 cup black beans, cooked and drained
1 cup kidney beans, cooked and drained
2 tablespoon hot sauce
¼ cup chopped cilantro

## Directions:

In a large saucepan over medium heat, heat the oil. Cook the onion until softened (approximately 3-4 minutes).

Add the garlic and cook for an additional 3 minutes.

Add the celery, chili powder, cumin, coriander and sea salt. Stir until combined.

Add the tomatoes, water and beans and bring to a boil. Reduce heat, cover and simmer for 20 minutes.

Add hot sauce to taste and garnish with cilantro.

Makes 4 servings

# Walnut Vinaigrette (dressing)

## Ingredients:

¼ cup extra virgin olive oil
¼ cup walnut pieces
2 tablespoons apple cider vinegar
1 teaspoon Dijon mustard
1 clove garlic
½ teaspoon sea salt
¼ teaspoon ground black pepper

## Directions:

Combine ingredients in a mini food processor or blender and blend till smooth.

Extra dressing can be stored for 3-5 days in the refrigerator. Shake well before using.

Makes approximately ½ cup

# White Balsamic Vinaigrette (dressing)

## Ingredients:

2 tablespoons white balsamic vinegar
½ cup extra virgin olive oil
½ teaspoon sea salt
¼ teaspoon ground black pepper

## Directions:

In a small stainless bowl, pour in the white balsamic vinegar. Slowly pour in the olive oil as you aggressively whisk until thoroughly combined. Add salt and pepper and whisk some more.

Store unused dressing in the refrigerator for 3-5 days.

Makes about 1 cup

# White Bean and Asparagus Salad*

## Ingredients:

1 bunch (12–16 spears) asparagus, trimmed and cut into 2" pieces
1 can (15 ounces) white beans, such as navy, rinsed and drained
6 grape tomatoes, halved
3 scallions, chopped
1/4 cup chopped fresh flat-leaf parsley
1/4 cup white balsamic vinegar
1 tablespoon extra-virgin olive oil
1 teaspoon Dijon mustard
1/4 teaspoon sea salt
1/4 teaspoon ground black pepper

## Directions:

In a medium saucepan with a steamer basket, bring 1" of water to a boil. Put the asparagus in the basket, cover, and steam for 3 to 5 minutes, or until tender. Do not overcook. Lift the asparagus from the steamer basket and let cool.

In a medium bowl, combine the beans, tomatoes, scallions, parsley, and cooled asparagus.

In a small bowl, whisk together the vinegar, oil, and mustard. Add the salt and pepper and whisk to combine. Pour the dressing over the bean salad and gently toss.

Makes 2 servings

*This recipe is from my Healthy You Diet cookbook. You can find out more or get the link to Amazon at* DawnaStone.com

# White Bean Hummus and Veggies (snack)

## Ingredients:

1 garlic clove, crushed

2 tablespoons Tahini sesame seed paste

2 tablespoons freshly squeezed lime juice

1 tablespoon extra virgin olive oil

¾ teaspoon salt

1 (15 oz) can navy beans rinsed and drained

2-4 tablespoons water (use more or less, based on desired consistency)

6 baby carrots

4 celery stalks, halved

½ cucumber, sliced

## Directions:

In food processor, combine garlic, tahini, lime juice, olive oil and salt. Blend for 30 seconds. Scrape mixture from sides of food processor. Add half the beans and blend for 1 minute. Scrape mixture from sides and add remaining beans. Add water for desired consistency. Serve with fresh vegetables. Cover and refrigerate any leftover hummus.

Makes 2 servings

# White Chicken Stew

## Ingredients:

2 tablespoons extra virgin olive oil
1 clove garlic, minced
1 yellow onion, chopped
2 ribs celery, chopped
1 large (or 3 small) carrots, peeled and chopped
Sea salt
Ground black pepper
1 yellow pepper, chopped
1 jalapeño, diced (optional)
½ Anaheim pepper, diced
1 can diced green chilies
6 cups chicken broth
1 cans northern beans
1 cup chopped kale
1 rotisserie chicken, boned, skinned and coarsely chopped

## Directions:

In a Dutch oven, heat the oil over medium-high heat. Add the garlic, onion, celery, and carrots. Sauté for approximately 5 minutes or until the onion is translucent. Add salt and pepper.

Add the yellow pepper, jalapeño, Anaheim pepper, and green

chilies and cook an additional 3-5 minutes. Add the broth, beans and kale. Bring to a boil, reduce the heat, and simmer for 25 minutes, or until the vegetables are tender. Add chicken and simmer an additional 5 to 10 minutes or until chicken is warmed through.

Makes 4 servings

# Bonus Recipes

These additional recipes are healthy and low in calories and can easily be helpful if you are developing your own meal plans.

# Breakfast Tacos

## Ingredients:

4 large eggs
4 corn tortillas
Olive oil spray
1 tablespoon diced onion
¼ cup tomato, diced
¼ jalapeño, diced
1 cup baby spinach, stems removed
¼ cup queso fresco, crumbled*
½ teaspoon salt
¼ teaspoon black pepper
Hot sauce, to taste (optional)

## Directions:

In a mixing bowl, whisk the eggs.

Lightly char each tortilla by placing them in a pan over medium high heat. Flip the tortilla often so it doesn't burn. Remove when tortilla begins to show light brown spots. Reserve tortillas.

Coat a medium skillet with olive oil spray. Add onion and cook for 1 to 2 minutes or until translucent. Add the tomato, jalapeño and spinach and cook for 1 minute or until spinach is wilted. Pour in the eggs and cook for 3 to 4 minutes or until desired doneness. Remove from heat.

Top the four tortillas with egg mixture. Add queso, salt, pepper and hot sauce (optional).

Makes 4 tacos

# Green Veggie Juice

## Ingredients:

1 cup baby spinach, stems removed
1 green apple, core removed
1 rib celery
½ cucumber
½ lemon
1-inch piece fresh ginger

## Directions:

In a juicer, juice the spinach, apple, celery, cucumber, lemon and ginger. Pour over ice and enjoy.

Makes 1 serving

# Vegetable Omelet

## Ingredients:

2 large eggs
2 teaspoon extra-virgin olive oil
1 tablespoon sweet onion, thinly chopped
1 small tomato, chopped
3 small button mushrooms, sliced
½ cup fresh baby spinach leaves, stems removed
¼ teaspoon sea salt
1/8 teaspoon black pepper

## Directions:

In a small bowl, whisk the eggs and set aside.

Coat a small nonstick skillet with 1 teaspoon olive oil and heat over medium heat.

Cook the onion for 1 minute or until translucent. Toss in the tomato and mushrooms and cook for an additional 4 to 5 minutes, or until tender. Transfer vegetables to a bowl.

Clean the skillet and coat with the remaining teaspoon of olive oil. Set over medium-high

heat. Add the reserved eggs and cook for 2 minutes (do not stir).

As the center sets, transfer the cooked vegetables to one side of the omelet. Top with the spinach. Season with salt and pepper. Gently fold 1 side of the omelet over the other.

Cook for 1 minute to let set. Remove from skillet and serve.

Makes 1 serving

# 21 Day IF Journal

# INTERMITTENT FASTING JOURNAL

Day

**Weight:**

**Breakfast:**

**Lunch:**

**Snack (optional):**

**Dinner:**

**Exercise:**

**Notes:**

# INTERMITTENT FASTING JOURNAL

Day

Weight:

Breakfast:

Lunch:

Snack (optional):

Dinner:

Exercise:

Notes:

# INTERMITTENT FASTING JOURNAL

Day

Weight:

Breakfast:

Lunch:

Snack (optional):

Dinner:

Exercise:

Notes:

# INTERMITTENT FASTING JOURNAL

Day

Weight:

Breakfast:

Lunch:

Snack (optional):

Dinner:

Exercise:

Notes:

# INTERMITTENT FASTING JOURNAL

Day

Weight:

Breakfast:

Lunch:

Snack (optional):

Dinner:

Exercise:

Notes:

# INTERMITTENT FASTING JOURNAL

Day

**Weight:**

**Breakfast:**

**Lunch:**

**Snack (optional):**

**Dinner:**

**Exercise:**

**Notes:**

# INTERMITTENT FASTING JOURNAL

Day

Weight:

Breakfast:

Lunch:

Snack (optional):

Dinner:

Exercise:

Notes:

# INTERMITTENT FASTING JOURNAL

Day

**Weight:**

**Breakfast:**

**Lunch:**

**Snack (optional):**

**Dinner:**

**Exercise:**

**Notes:**

# INTERMITTENT FASTING
## JOURNAL

Day

Weight:

Breakfast:

Lunch:

Snack (optional):

Dinner:

Exercise:

Notes:

# INTERMITTENT FASTING
## JOURNAL

Day

Weight:

Breakfast:

Lunch:

Snack (optional):

Dinner:

Exercise:

Notes:

# INTERMITTENT FASTING JOURNAL

**Day**

**Weight:**

**Breakfast:**

**Lunch:**

**Snack (optional):**

**Dinner:**

**Exercise:**

**Notes:**

# INTERMITTENT FASTING JOURNAL

Day

Weight:

Breakfast:

Lunch:

Snack (optional):

Dinner:

Exercise:

Notes:

# INTERMITTENT FASTING
# JOURNAL

Day

Weight:

Breakfast:

Lunch:

Snack (optional):

Dinner:

Exercise:

Notes:

# INTERMITTENT FASTING JOURNAL

Day

Weight:

Breakfast:

Lunch:

Snack (optional):

Dinner:

Exercise:

Notes:

# INTERMITTENT FASTING JOURNAL

| Day |
| --- |

**Weight:**

**Breakfast:**

**Lunch:**

**Snack (optional):**

**Dinner:**

**Exercise:**

**Notes:**

# INTERMITTENT FASTING JOURNAL

Day

Weight:

Breakfast:

Lunch:

Snack (optional):

Dinner:

Exercise:

Notes:

# INTERMITTENT FASTING JOURNAL

Day

**Weight:**

Breakfast:

Lunch:

Snack (optional):

Dinner:

Exercise:

Notes:

# INTERMITTENT FASTING JOURNAL

Day

Weight:

Breakfast:

Lunch:

Snack (optional):

Dinner:

Exercise:

Notes:

# INTERMITTENT FASTING JOURNAL

Day

**Weight:**

Breakfast:

Lunch:

Snack (optional):

Dinner:

Exercise:

Notes:

# INTERMITTENT FASTING
# JOURNAL

Day

Weight:

Breakfast:

Lunch:

Snack (optional):

Dinner:

Exercise:

Notes:

# INTERMITTENT FASTING JOURNAL

Day

Weight:

Breakfast:

Lunch:

Snack (optional):

Dinner:

Exercise:

Notes:

# Endnotes

1. Albata, K. (2014). Fasting in world history (UC Berkeley). YouTube.com. Retrieved from https://www.youtube.com/watch?v=OD5Nhv18JKs

2. Polar Light Organization. (2019). The history of fasting. Retrieved from http://www.polarlight.org/the-history-of-fasting.html

3. Ibid.

4. Ibid.

5. Link, R. (2018). 8 Health Benefits of Fasting, Backed by Science. Heathline.com. Retrieved from https://www.healthline.com/nutrition/fasting-benefits#section1

6. Bhupathiraju, Shilpa N., and Frank B. Hu. "Epidemiology of obesity and diabetes and their cardiovascular complications." *Circulation research* 118, no. 11 (2016): 1723-1735.

7. BBC. (2012). Horizons: Eat, Fast and Live Longer. Retrieved from https://www.bbc.co.uk/programmes/b011xyzc

8. Harvie, Michelle N., Mary Pegington, Mark P. Mattson, Jan Frystyk, Bernice Dillon, Gareth Evans, Jack Cuzick et al. "The effects of intermittent or continuous energy restriction on weight loss and metabolic disease risk markers: a randomized trial in young overweight women." *International journal of obesity* 35, no. 5 (2011): 714.

9. Mosley, Michael. *The Fast Diet–Revised & Updated: Lose Weight, Stay Healthy, and Live Longer with the Simple Secret of Intermittent Fasting.* New York: Atria Paperback, 2015.

10. Longo, Valter D., and Mark P. Mattson. "Fasting: molecular mechanisms and clinical applications." *Cell metabolism* 19, no. 2 (2014): 181-192.

11. Ibid.

12. Patterson, Ruth E., Gail A. Laughlin, Andrea Z. LaCroix, Sheri J. Hartman, Loki Natarajan, Carolyn M. Senger, María Elena Martínez et al. "Intermittent fasting and human metabolic health." *Journal of the Academy of Nutrition and Dietetics* 115, no. 8 (2015): 1203-1212.

13. Ibid.

14. Ibid.

15. Ibid.

16. Ibid.

17. Stockman, Mary-Catherine, Dylan Thomas, Jacquelyn Burke, and Caroline M. Apovian. "Intermittent fasting: is the wait worth the weight?" *Current obesity reports* 7 (2018): 172-185.

18. Patterson, 2015.

19. Ibid.

20. Ibid.

21. Ibid.

22. Patterson, Ruth E., Gail A. Laughlin, Andrea Z. LaCroix, Sheri J. Hartman, Loki Natarajan, Carolyn M. Senger, María Elena Martínez et al. "Intermittent fasting and human metabolic health." *Journal of the Academy of Nutrition and Dietetics* 115, no. 8 (2015): 1203-1212.

23. Ibid.

24. Ibid.

25. Stockman, Mary-Catherine, Dylan Thomas, Jacquelyn Burke, and Caroline M. Apovian. "Intermittent fasting: is the wait worth the weight?" *Current obesity reports* 7 (2018): 172-185.

26. Patterson, 2015.

27. Ibid.

28. Ibid.

29. Ibid.

30. Barnosky, A. R., Hoddy, K. K., Unterman, T. G., & Varady, K. A. (2014). Intermittent fasting vs daily calorie restriction for type 2 diabetes prevention: a review of human findings. *Translational Research, 164*(4), 302-311.

31. Longo, V. D., & Mattson, M. P. (2014). Fasting: molecular mechanisms and clinical applications. *Cell metabolism, 19*(2), 181-192.

32. Ibid.

33. Varady, K. A. (2011). Intermittent versus daily calorie restriction: which diet regimen is more effective for weight loss? *Obesity reviews, 12*(7), e593-e601.

34. Barnosky, 2014.

35. Varady, 2011.

36. Longo, V. D., & Mattson, M. P. (2014). Fasting: molecular mechanisms and clinical applications. *Cell metabolism, 19*(2), 181-192.

37. BBC. (2012). Horizons: Eat, Fast and Live Longer. Retrieved from https://www.bbc.co.uk/programmes/b01lxyzc

38. Barnosky, Adrienne R., Kristin K. Hoddy, Terry G. Unterman, and Krista A. Varady. "Intermittent fasting vs daily calorie restriction for type 2 diabetes prevention: a review of human findings." *Translational Research* 164, no. 4 (2014): 302-311.

CPSIA information can be obtained
at www.ICGtesting.com
Printed in the USA
BVHW042052010120
568277BV00016B/900/P